POULTRY DISEASES
UNDER
MODERN MANAGEMENT

(Second Edition)

by

G.S. COUTTS B.V.M.S., M.R.C.V.S.

Published by
SAIGA PUBLISHING CO., LTD
1 ROYAL PARADE, HINDHEAD
SURREY GU26 6TD ENGLAND

First edition published for *Poultry World* 1960.
Second, fully revised, edition 1981.

Typesetting by Inforum Ltd.
Printed and bound by
Robert Hartnoll Ltd., Bodmin, Cornwall.
Published by
SAIGA PUBLISHING CO. LTD.,
1 Royal Parade, Hindhead, Surrey GU26 6TD, England.

Contents

LIST OF MONOCHROME ILLUSTRATIONS

LIST OF COLOURED PLATES

Plate

1   Internal Organs of the Fowl

2   Avian Tuberculosis
Aspergills fumigatus
Caecal Coccidiosis
Blackhead

3   Gangrenous dermatitis
Erysipelas
Infectious synovitis
Mycoplasma gallisepticum infection

4   Infectious bursal disease – haemorrhages in breast and thigh
muscles
Infectious bursal disease – inflammation of cloacal bursa
Infectious bursal disease – haemorrhages in proventriculus
Inclusion-body hepatitis

5   Colisepticaemia
Marek's disease – nodular lesions in liver
Marek's disease – enlargement of vagus nerve in neck
Lymphoid leucosis

6   Slipped tendon
Ruptured tendon
Plantar pododermatisis
Articular gout

7   Gizzard impaction
Sour crop
Volvulus or twisted gut
Staphylococcal arthritis

8   Swelling and pallor of kidneys
Fatty liver haemorrhagic syndrome
Round heart disease
Gizzard erosion

Introduction

In the introduction to the first edition of this book in 1961, it was mentioned that important changes were taking place in the poultry industry, particularly that intensivism within the industry was gaining momentum. The free range system was being replaced by the cage laying unit and an enormous expansion of broiler growing was taking place. Since that time, these trends have continued to the extent that over 95 per cent of eggs are now produced by caged layers. Still larger broiler units now accommodate 20,000 or more birds per house, and 100,000 or more per site.

When it is considered that this vast multi-million-pound industry has evolved in the space of little more than twenty years from a 'backyard' system of poultry keeping which did little more than provide pin-money for the farmer's wife, it may be scarcely surprising that the growth of the industry has been accompanied by a good many problems associated with environment, husbandry and disease.

It is the purpose of this book to present a brief account of the most important poultry diseases in a form which, it is hoped, will be intelligible to the layman who has an interest in poultry keeping and also wishes to know a little about the diseases from which his birds may suffer, their main signs and post-mortem changes, treatment, prevention and so on.

The book is intended only as an *introduction* to poultry disease. Larger, more detailed volumes are available to those who require a deeper knowledge of the subject. While it is impossible to avoid a certain number of technical names and terms, it is hoped that these have been kept to an acceptable minimum.

The subject matter has been restricted to a description of the main poultry diseases as they occur under modern management conditions. Actual descriptions of management and husbandry practices, nutrition, etc., have been omitted, as these will be found in a companion volume — *Practical Poultry Keeping* by John Portsmouth (Saiga Publishing).

CHAPTER 1

Identifying the Diseases

INTRODUCTION

Diseases are normally classified on the basis of origin or cause:

1. Bacterial
2. Viral
3. Parasitic
4. Leg Diseases
5. Miscellaneous

This is the procedure adopted in this book and readers are advised to study the Contents List to see the heading under which each disease falls. Inevitably there is some overlap particularly with the miscellaneous and leg diseases which may also be bacterial, viral or parasitic to some extent.

For the purpose of locating the possible nature of a disease as quickly as possible, the following pages show the **principal diseases**, the **main species affected**, **likely age**, **signs**, **treatment** and **page** where further details may be found.

The **Diagnostic Disease Chart** is arranged alphabetically, so no difficulty should be experienced in locating a specific disease. However, the descriptions in the chart are necessarily brief and careful checking with the appropriate chapter will be essential before forming a final conclusion. In many cases a post mortem examination may be essential, especially when serious mortality or outbreaks have occurred.

1

DIAGNOSTIC DISEASES CHART

DISEASE	MAIN SPECIES AFFECTED	LIKELY AGE (in weeks where no. specified)	SIGNS	TREATMENT	Page Ref.
Ammonia blindness	Chicken	Over 6	Eye irritation; closed eyes; conjunctivitis; rubbing eyes on wings; frosted glass appearance of eye	Reduce ammonia levels by attention to litter and ventilation	219
Aortic rupture	Turkey	Over 10	None. Sudden death	None: prevent by including *Reserpine* (sedative) in food	225
Arizona infection	Turkey	Up to 3	Dejection; inappetance; diarrhoea; nervous signs; blindness	*Furazolidone*; *Furaltadone*	66
Aspergillosis	Chicken, Turkey Duck	Up to 3, sometimes older birds	Inappetance; weakness; silent gasping; variable mortality	None	145
Avian encephalomyelitis (epidemic tremor)	Chicken	Baby chicks, layers	A. Baby chicks – nervous signs; imbalance; chicks off legs, lying on sides; tremors of head, neck and wings; some mortality. B. Layers – sharp drop in egg production	None: prevent by vaccination	98
Biotin deficiency	Turkey	4–10	Poor growth; leg weakness; scabs around eyes and corners of beak; thickened skin on undersides of feet	Addition of *biotin* to diet	190
Blackhead	Turkeys – occasionally Chicken Pheasants	4–12, occasionally older	Depression; inappetance; poor growth; sulphur-yellow diarrhoea; variable mortality	*Dimetridazole*: also used for prevention in food	164
Botulism	Waterfowl Chickens	All ages, mainly broilers and waterfowl over 4	Nervous signs; weakness; progressive paralysis of neck, wings and legs; death from respiratory paralysis	None: remove source of toxin	56

Disease	Species	Age (weeks)	Signs	Treatment	Page
Caecal worm	Chicken Turkey	Over 3	None	*Levamisole*: treatment not usually required	175
Coccidiosis	All species	2–6, also older birds	Signs depend on type of coccidiosis, include depression; ruffled feathers; closed eyes; loss of appetite; poor growth; diarrhoea; blood in droppings; variable mortality	*Sulphonamides*: including *Sulphamezathine*; *Sulphaquinoxaline*; also *amprolium* and other drugs; prevent by *coccidiostats* in feed	151
Colisepticaemia	Chicken Turkey Duck	4–8	Respiratory signs; coughing; sneezing; dejection; reduced appetite; poor growth; variable mortality	Antibiotics; *Furazolidone*; *Furaltadone*	42
Duck virus enteritis	Duck Goose	Any age	Depression; loss of appetite; thirst; discharge from eyes and nostrils; imbalance; diarrhoea, sometimes with blood	None: prevention by vaccination (USA)	139
Duck virus hepatitis	Duck	Under 3	Depression; birds fall on sides; paddling movements of legs; arching of back; very rapid death	None: prevent by vaccination or anti-serum (USA)	136
Egg drop syndrome 1976	Chicken	Layers at peak production	Egg drop at peak production or failure to peak; soft shelled and shell-less eggs	None: prevent by vaccination	118
Erysipelas	Turkey	Over 6	Inappetance; depression; diarrhoea; snood swollen; rapid death	*Penicillin*	63
Fatty liver and kidney syndrome	Chicken	2–6	Depression; reduced appetite; slight inco-ordination; variable mortality	Add *biotin* to food or water or molasses to water	217
Fatty liver haemorrhagic syndrome	Chicken	Birds in lay	Birds overweight; sudden death usually with no preceding signs	Reduce flock's energy intake	214

3

DIAGNOSTIC DISEASES CHART

DISEASE	MAIN SPECIES AFFECTED	LIKELY AGE (in weeks where no. specified)	SIGNS	TREATMENT	Page Ref.
Favus	Chicken Turkey	Mainly adults	White, powdery spots or wrinkled crusts and scab on comb and wattles; loss of feathers; thick crusty skin; loss of condition	Remove crusts; apply ointment of *formalin* in petroleum jelly	149
Fowl Plague	Chicken Turkey	Any age	Depression; coughing; discharge from eyes and nostrils; swollen face; diarrhoea; nervous signs; paralysis	None: slaugter with compensation (UK)	140
Fowl Pox	Chicken Turkey	Any age, mainly adults	Warty, spreading eruptions on comb and wattles; caseous deposits in mouth and throat; depression; inappetance; poor egg production	None: prevent by vaccination	108
Fowl Typhoid	Chicken Turkey Duck	Point of lay pullets, adults	Dejection; ruffled feathers; inappetance; thirst; reluctance to move; yellow diarrhoea; severe emaciation; high mortality	*Furazolidone; Furaltadone*	17
Gangrenous dermatitis	Chickens	4–8	Usually no signs; occasionally dejection; loss of appetite; rapid death	*Sulphaquinoxaline;* antibiotics; *Tetracyclines; Penicillin*	56, 8
Gapeworm	Pheasant Chicken Turkey	3–12, occasionally older birds	Gaping; gasping; difficult breathing; loss of appetite and condition; some mortality	*Gapex; Mebenvet Thiabendazole*	175
Gizzard worm	Goose	Goslings 3–12, occasionally older birds	Depression; loss of condition and weight; slow growth; some mortality	*Levamisole*	175

4

Disease	Species	Age (weeks)	Symptoms	Treatment	Page
Haemorrhagic disease	Chicken	4–8 or older	Dejection; loss of appetite; poor growth; pale comb and wattles; blood in droppings	Vitamin K in water: remove or reduce *sulphonamides* where used	228
Hairworm	Chicken	Over 4	Loss of condition; slow growth; listlessness; diarrhoea; some mortality	*Levamisole*	175
Hexamitiasis	Turkey Pheasant	2–6 or 8, occasionally older	Depression; inappetance; loss of weight; frothy, watery-yellow droppings; often high mortality	*Furazolidone; Tetracycline;* antibiotics; *Dimetridazole*	169
Inclusion body hepatitis	Chicken	5–7	Depression; ruffled feathers; inappetance; rapid death	None	116
Infectious bronchitis	Chicken	Any age	A. Chicks and growers – depression; huddling; loss of appetite; coughing; gasping; difficult breathing. B. Layers – loss of egg production; soft shelled eggs; rough shells	No specific treatment: antibiotics to control secondary infection: prevent by vaccination	88
Infectious Bursal disease (Gumboro disease)	Chicken	2–6	Depression; inappetance; unsteady gait; pecking at vent; diarrhoea	None: prevent by vaccination	102
Infectious Coryza	Chicken	Adults	Facial swelling; ocular and nasal discharge; sneezing; difficult breathing; loss of condition and egg production; inappetance; variable mortality	Antibiotics	67
Infectious laryngotracheitis	Chicken Pheasant	Over 6	Difficult breathing; gasping; coughing of mucus or blood; rapid death; loss of egg production	No specific treatment: antibiotics to control secondary infection: prevent by vaccination	94

DIAGNOSTIC DISEASES CHART

DISEASE	MAIN SPECIES AFFECTED	LIKELY AGE (in weeks where no. specified)	SIGNS	TREATMENT	Page Ref.
Lice	Chicken Turkey	Maily adults	Irritation; loss of vent feathers; scabs around vent; loss of condition and egg production	*BHC, pyrethrum* etc., dusting powders; *Organophosphorus* sprays	178
Lymphoid leucosis	Chicken	Over 16	No paralysis; depression; loss of weight; emaciation; variable mortality	None	131
Manganese deficiency (Perosis)	Chicken Turkey	Unhatched embryos, growing birds	Short legs; parrot beak and other deformities of embryo; high dead-in-shell; lameness; distortion of hock; slipping of achilles tendon from hock	Addition of manganese to diet	197
Marek's disease	Chicken	Over 6	Paralysis of legs, wings, neck; depression; loss of weight; variable mortality	None: prevent by vaccination	122
Moniliasis	Chicken Turkey	Young poults and chicks	Dejection; poor appetite; slow growth	*Mycostatin*; copper sulphate (value doubtful)	149
Mycoplasma gallisepticum infection	Chicken Turkey	Over 4	Coughing; nasal discharge; watery eyes; swollen sinuses; slow growth; leg problems; stunting	Antibiotics; *Erythromycin; Tylosin; Spiramycin*	71
Mycoplasma meleagridis infection	Turkey	Over 4	Coughing; sneezing; slow growth; stunting; leg problems	Antibiotics; *Tylosin; Erythromycin; Spiramycin*	77
Mycoplasma synoviae infection (Infectious synovitis)	Chicken Turkey	Over 4	Depression; inappetance; ruffled feathers; lameness; birds off legs; swelling on hocks, shanks and feet	Antibiotics; *Chlortetracycline*	74

Disease	Species	Age (weeks)	Signs	Treatment/Prevention	Page
Mycotoxicosis	Chicken Turkey Duck	Any age, mainly growers	Signs variable; include poor growth; depression; diarrhoea; blood in droppings; thirst; loss of egg production; poor feathering	Remove source of toxin by replacing food, litter	220
Necrotic enteritis	Chicken	Over 6 up to point of lay; occasionally birds in lay	Depression; ruffled feathers; inappetance; closed eyes; reluctance to move; dark coloured diarrhoea	*Penicillin*	60
Newcastle disease	Chicken Turkey Also other species	Any age	Depression; inappetance; coughing; difficult breathing; diarrhoea; nervous signs; paralysis; twisted necks; drop in egg production	No specific treatment: antibiotics to control secondary infection: prevent by vaccination	81
Nutritional encephalomalacia (Crazy chick disease, Vitamin E deficiency)	Chicken	Up to 5	Imbalance; staggering; uncontrolled movements; falling over; somersaults; twisted neck; paralysis; variable mortality	Addition of Vitamin E to diet	195
Oedema syndrome	Turkey	4–14 days	Sudden death	Attend to management; reduce food intake	228
Pasteurellosis (Fowl cholera)	Chicken Turkey	Chicken – mainly adults; Turkey – over 8	Dejection; ruffled feathers; loss of appetite; diarrhoea; coughing; discharge from nostrils, eyes, mouth; swollen wattles; lameness; sudden death; variable mortality	*Sulphaquinoxaline* antibiotics	47
Pullet disease	Chicken	16–40	Depression; loss of appetite; crop distension; dark comb and wattles; diarrhoea; drop in egg production	Adequate water supply; antibiotics; molasses in water	230

7

DIAGNOSTIC DISEASES CHART

DISEASE	MAIN SPECIES AFFECTED	LIKELY AGE (in weeks where no. specified)	SIGNS	TREATMENT	Page Ref.
Pullorum disease	Chicken Turkey	Up to 3	Inappetance; depression; ruffled feathers; closed eyes; loud chirping; white diarrhoea; vent pasting; gasping; lameness; high mortality	*Furazolidone; Furaltadone*	11
Red Mite	Chicken Turkey	Mainly adults	Irritation; restlessness; loss of condition; pale comb and wattles; loss of egg production	*BHC; Pyrethrum* etc., dusting powders; *Organophosphorus* sprays	181
Riboflavin deficiency	Chicken Turkey	Unhatched embryo, baby chicks and poults	High dead-in-shells; clubbed down; curled toes; poor growth	Addition of riboflavin to diet	189
Rickets (Vitamin D deficiency, calcium or phosphorus deficiency or imbalance)	Chicken Turkey Duck	2–6	Lameness; hock swelling; soft bones and beak; many birds go off legs suddenly	Addition of Vitamin D, calcium or phosphorus to diet	191
Roundworm (large)	All species	Over 4	Loss of condition; slow growth; listlessness; diarrhoea	*Piperazine; Levamisole*	175
Round heart disease	Chicken Turkey	8–20	Sudden death; depression; inappetance; blue comb and wattles	Add vitamins to water; change food; remove litter	226
Ruptured gastrocnemius tendon	Broiler Chicken	Over 7, capons and roasters	Severe lameness; hock rests on floor; green discoloration of the tissues around hock	None	204

8

Disease	Species	Age affected (weeks)	Symptoms	Treatment	Page
Salmonellosis	Chicken Turkey Duck	Baby chicks and poults up to 3	Dejection; ruffled feathers; closed eyes; diarrhoea; vent pasting; loss of appetite; thirst; high mortality	*Furazolidone; Furaltadone*	24
Scaly leg	Chicken Turkey	Mainly adults	Irritation; lameness; raised, distorted leg scales; crusty masses on legs	Dip legs in paraffin, *BHC* and other insecticidal emulsions	180
Shaky leg syndrome	Turkey	Over 8	Shaking or quivering of legs when bird rises after resting	None	205
Spondylolisthesis (Kinky back)	Broiler chicken	4 and over	Sitting on rump with legs extended in front, supported by wings; bird moves backwards when attempting to walk	None	203
Spraddle legs	All species	Baby chicks	Legs splay out and chick is unable to stand	None	206
Staphylococcal arthritis (Bumblefoot)	Chicken Turkey	Growers; pullets up to point of lay	Lameness; reluctance to move; swollen hocks and feet	Antibiotics	52
Tibial dyschondroplasia	Turkey Duck Chicken	5–8	Lameness; reluctance to move; swelling and bowing of bones in region of knee joint	None	200
Tuberculosis	Chicken	Adults; old birds	Severe loss of weight without loss of appetite; pale comb; diarrhoea; lameness; occasional deaths	None	32
Twisted leg	Chicken Turkey	Over 2	Lameness; distortion at hock; various angulations of affected leg	None	202
Vibrionic hepatitis	Chicken	Over 16	Dejection; diarrhoea; loss of condition; inappetance; pale comb and wattles; variable mortality	*Furazolidone;* antibiotics	68

DIAGNOSTIC DISEASES CHART

DISEASE	MAIN SPECIES AFFECTED	LIKELY AGE (in weeks where no. specified)	SIGNS	TREATMENT	Page Ref.
Viral arthritis	Chicken	5–8 or older	Lameness; reluctance to move; poor growth; inflammation around hock	None	199
Vitamin A deficiency (Nutritional Roup)	Chicken Turkey	Any age, mainly adults	Loss of condition; poor feathering; discharge from eyes and nostrils; difficult breathing; eyelids stuck together; pale comb and wattles; pustules in mouth	Addition of Vitamin A to food	188
Yolk sac infection	Chicken Turkey Duck	Baby chicks and poults under 1	Dejection; closed eyes; loss of appetite; diarrhoea; vent pasting; swollen abdomen; increased mortality in 1st week	Antibiotics; *Furazolidone; Furaltadone*	36

NOTE: Reference should be made to the illustrations of the main diseases.

CHAPTER 2

Pullorum disease

BACKGROUND

Pullorum disease or **bacillary white diarrhoea** was first described in 1900 as being caused by a member of the Salmonella group of bacteria, *Salmonella pullorum*. It was quickly recognised as one of the most serious menaces that threatened the poultry industry. Since then it has been found to occur in practically all parts of the world in which poultry are kept and, because of its great incidence, it has been studied extensively so as to devise effective methods of control. As a result, the disease has been almost eliminated from Britain and a number of other countries in which control methods have been rigorously applied. However, if the poultry industries of these countries are to remain free of infection there can be no relaxation of vigilance. The disease still occurs widely in poultry in less advanced areas of the world.

Primarily a disease of chicks, pullorum disease also occurs in turkey poults and outbreaks have been reported in pheasants. Ducklings and goslings are rather resistant to infection and the disease is of little importance in these species. *Salmonella pullorum* also occurs in wild birds but there is little evidence that it gives rise to outbreaks of disease.

SOURCE OF INFECTION

After an outbreak of pullorum disease has occurred surviving chicks may become carriers of infection, i.e. the *Salmonella pullorum* bacteria are not completely eliminated from the body but remain localised in the bird's internal organs for long periods, often for life. The organ in which infection most commonly remains is the ovary, and although the bird may show no signs of ill health the organism infects a proportion of the eggs laid. If these eggs hatch the chicks that emerge will develop pullorum disease. It only requires one or two infected chicks to set up a severe outbreak in the remainder of the hatch, since they eliminate large numbers of organisms into the environment. Chick fluff is particularly dangerous because, as soon as it is dry, it, and the bacteria it contains are dispersed rapidly throughout the incubator or hatcher by air currents. Other chicks may become infected by swallowing this material or by inhaling it, when the organism gives rise to a highly fatal form of pneumonia.

There are other methods whereby pullorum disease can be transmitted; e.g., by contamination of the eggshell with infected faeces from a carrier bird, or by ingestion of contaminated feed or water, which can occur in birds of any age. These, however, are of minor importance compared with eggborne transmission from a bird with an infected ovary. Pullorum disease was in fact one of the first diseases in which transmission via the hatching egg was definitely established.

Most chicks that survive pullorum disease become carriers of infection. The number of infected eggs laid by carrier hens varies considerably, but it is usually in the region of 5 to 10 per cent of total production.

Although carrier hens in infected flocks generally appear healthy their egg production tends to be lower than that of non-infected birds, probably by about 10 to 20 per cent. The fertility and hatchability of their eggs is also reduced. Thus carrier birds may not only give rise to outbreaks of pullorum disease; they are also a much poorer financial proposition.

SIGNS AND COURSE OF DISEASE

In acute outbreaks chicks may die from pullorum disease without showing any signs of ill health. In less acute cases there is loss of vigour, sluggishness, drooped wings and ruffled feathers. Appetite is lost. Chicks huddle together and chirp loudly, or stand alone looking dejected with closed eyes. A white diarrhoea is frequently present and this may give rise to vent pasting. Eventually there is extreme weakness and chicks may be found lying on their sides shortly before death.

In cases in which lung lesions are present, gasping and difficulty in breathing may occur while severe lameness will be present in cases in which the joints are affected.

These signs are not sufficiently characteristic to distinguish pullorum disease from other forms of Salmonella infection, or indeed from other diseases of chicks. Post mortem and bacteriological examinations are therefore necessary to establish a diagnosis.

In most outbreaks highest mortality occurs between five and ten days post–hatching, suggesting that infection was egg transmitted and disseminated in the incubator. In other cases when infection is picked up later, losses start later with peak mortality occurring possibly as late as two to three weeks of age. Generally however resistance to infection increases with age so that by the time chicks are ten days to two weeks old they may be difficult to infect, and in those that do become infected the disease takes a mild form with a low death rate. Chicks that survive the acute form of the disease make a slow recovery, but it may be a long time before their condition approaches that of uninfected birds and some birds never fully recover.

There also occurs a chronic form of pullorum disease in which mortality is low but in which chicks show general unthriftiness and lameness at two to five weeks of age. It may be that birds suffering from this form of the disease are, in reality, survivors of an outbreak which occurred when the birds were a few days old.

Apart from age there are a number of factors that have an adverse effect on the death rate that may be experienced in any particular outbreak. These include poor hygiene, overcrowding, certain dietary deficiencies and the presence of other diseases normally of only slight significance. Chilling from draughty, cold conditions experienced during transport or from incorrectly operated heating equipment may markedly increase the death rate.

It has also been shown that certain breeds of chicks are more resistant to pullorum disease than others. For example, chicks of the White Leghorn variety are in general more resistant than heavy breeds.

Only very occasionally is *Salmonella pullorum* responsible for deaths in adult birds. It is believed that in many cases where adults do succumb to the disease, they have survived attacks as chicks. Before death these adult birds lose condition, the comb and wattles become pale, diarrhoea may develop and they become progressively thinner. Usually only a small number of adults in a flock are affected by the disease, in contrast to the situation in chick flocks.

Post Mortem Findings

In chicks dying of the acute form of pullorum disease there may be no visible changes although the lungs or liver may be congested. In less acute cases the liver is enlarged with scattered foci of necrosis and is often of a dark mahogany colour. The heart is sometimes irregularly shaped due to multiple nodules scattered over its surface and similar nodules may be present in the lungs. Occasionally caseous casts are present in the caecal tubes. The contents of the yolk sac may be inspissated and flocculent or may be totally liquified.

In the joint form of the disease a gelatinous exudate is found in the joints and necrotic foci are often present in the liver and heart.

In adult birds suffering from or carrying pullorum disease characteristic changes are present in the ovaries. The ova are cyst-like in appearance and instead of being spherical they are grossly mis-shapen and are often attached to the ovary by long stalks. They have a rather "cooked" appearance, their walls being thickened and containing yellow strands inter-mingled with yellow, oily material. The livers of such birds are often enlarged and greenish-yellow in colour.

Diagnosis

Signs and post mortem changes are not sufficiently characteristic to enable a diagnosis to be made. In particular the disease cannot readily be distinguished from other Salmonella infections.

Bacteriological examination of the liver to isolate *Salmonella pullorum* is necessary for definitive diagnosis. In adult birds blood testing will detect flock infection, but again this should be confirmed by bacteriological examination of the heart, liver, spleen, ovary or other visibly affected tissues.

Identification of *Salmonella pullorum* and its differentiation from *Salmonella gallinarum* may be matters of some difficulty and tissues should be submitted to a well equipped laboratory for this purpose.

Treatment

Furazolidone or **furaltadone** are the drugs of choice for treating pullorum disease in young chicks. These drugs give good control of the infection and in most cases few carriers remain after treatment, although it is impossible to be sure that all have been eliminated. Furazolidone is generally used in the feed at a level of 0.04 per cent for ten days. Furaltadone, being more soluble is the drug of choice where water medication is to be used.

Breeding flocks found to be affected by pollorum disease should not be treated with a view to continued production of eggs for hatching, as some carrier birds may remain after treatment. Such flocks should be culled or the eggs sold commercially. Infected commercial, egg producing flocks may be treated and good control of the disease achieved.

PREVENTION AND CONTROL

While a large measure of control can be achieved by maintaining high standards of hygiene, cleanliness and sanitation in supply flocks, hatcheries and commercial poultry plants, the main method of controlling B.W.D. consists in ensuring that breeding flocks do not contain birds that are carriers. This is achieved by blood-testing of all birds in the breeding flock and eliminating those that give a positive reaction to the test, i.e., those that are found to be carriers of the infection. In Britain this is carried out under the Poultry Health Scheme of the Ministry of Agriculture.

The principle of the test is that when birds become infected with *Salmonella pullorum* they develop antibodies to the organism in their blood. When blood containing these antibodies is mixed with suspensions of *Salmonella pullorum* bacteria, instead of remaining as an even suspension, these bacteria aggregate together in clumps which are easily visible to the naked eye. The actual test may be carried out in tubes or, more commonly, on a white plate or tile. For the plate test, one of the wing veins of a chicken is pricked with a needle and a drop of blood is taken and mixed on the plate with a drop of a thick suspension of dead *Salmonella pullorum* bacteria that has been produced in the laboratory.

Mixing is facilitated by rotating the plate to and fro for a few moments and the test is read. Reading is facilitated by the fact that the bacteria have, during preparation in the laboratory, been coloured with a purple or violet dye. If the bacterial suspension remains even and homogeneous, the reaction is considered to be negative and this, of course, is indicative of a healthy bird. On the other hand, the aggregation of the bacteria into large purple clumps or granules indicates that the blood contained antibodies to *Salmonella pullorum* and, therefore, must have been taken from an infected bird. The test is know as the **whole blood, stained antigen, rapid plate agglutination test.** It may be carried out on the farm so that infected birds can be detected and eliminated immediately.

This testing of breeding flocks has now been rigidly applied in Britain for a number of years and has so reduced egg transmission of the disease that it may be regarded as almost totally eliminated from Britain. Fowl typhoid, which is detected by the same test, has been similarly eliminated.

CHAPTER 3

Fowl Typhoid

NATURE OF DISEASE

Fowl typhoid is a disease of poultry caused by the bacterial organism *Salmonella gallinarum* a member of the Salmonella group. Other Salmonella types produce their most serious effects in chicks, but *Salmonella gallinarum* is unique in that the greatest losses experienced under natural conditions are among adult birds.

Salmonella gallinarum closely resembles *Salmonella pullorum* (the cause of pullorum disease) in many ways, for in both cases exactly the same kind of antibodies are produced in the blood of infected birds. Consequently, the blood test for the detection of carriers of *Salmonella pullorum* employed in pullorum disease control projects applies equally well in the detection of birds which are carriers of fowl typhoid. At one time it was thought *Salmonella pullorum* and *Salmonella gallinarum* were identical, but it has now been clearly shown that while they do in fact have much in common they differ in a few important respects.

Fowl typhoid is probably one of the oldest diseases of poultry. It was first recognised in Britain in 1889 and has since been reported from most parts of the world. In Britain fowl typhoid was restricted largely to certain well-defined areas of Central Wales, the Western Midlands and the Western Islands of Scotland. The generally accepted view was that in these areas it was related to rather unprogressive methods of management and poor hygiene. For a time it became rather common in various other areas, but due to control methods it is now a rare disease in this country.

In other countries fowl typhoid may still be an important cause of loss in poultry flocks, particularly in warm, wet areas including parts of Africa. In America it was formerly rather common in turkeys, but in Britain it was rarely seen in this species.

SPECIES SUSCEPTIBLE

Chickens and turkeys are mainly affected, although ducks, geese, guinea fowl, pheasants, partridges, grouse, quail and pigeons may contract the disease. The causal organism has been found in certain wild birds such as rooks and sparrows.

As mentioned previously, fowl typhoid occurs mainly in adult birds, pullets coming into lay being most commonly affected. Most outbreaks have occurred in free range flocks, but when the disease gains entry to deep litter flocks it spreads rapidly and causes heavy losses. Most layers are now kept in battery cages and although the disease might be expected to spread more slowly under this system, severe outbreaks can also occur in caged birds, particularly where the disease has been egg transmitted. It may be that in some of these cases the disease has been present while the birds were being reared on litter but only becomes a serious problem when the flock is moved to laying cages, the birds then being at the age when most cases occur.

Outbreaks may be seen at all times of the year, but they are most common in the summer months, particularly if the weather is wet.

Signs

The first warning of an outbreak may be the sudden death of several birds which previously had shown no signs of ill health. Usually, however, birds are noted to be obviously ill for a few days before death. Affected birds appear thoroughly dejected with their feathers ruffled, head sunk on breast and wings drooping. They are reluctant to move about and stand motionless for long periods with one or both eyes closed. Their appetite is poor but their thirst, if anything, is increased. A very fluid yellow or greenish-yellow diarrhoea is a constant symptom of the disease. Most deaths take place within two to eight days of the onset of symptoms.

Birds that survive this period enter the chronic phase of the disease from which they may either die or make a slow recovery, the great majority of deaths from this form occurring within three to four weeks of contracting the disease. The main additional signs of the chronic disease are a severe progressive emaciation and an intense anaemia, the birds becoming extremely thin and the comb and wattles becoming yellowish-white and bloodless in appearance.

The number of birds in a flock that become ill, and the number that die, varies greatly from outbreak to outbreak. In some cases only a few birds contract the disease with few deaths, while in others all the birds in the flock may become infected, and as many as 80 to 90 per cent die. There are a number of factors which are known to have an important bearing on these points. Some of the factors which increase the severity of an outbreak are poor standards of hygiene and sanitation, overcrowding and damp weather conditions in birds running out of doors.

Diet also plays an important part and, strangely enough, the disease is usually more severe in birds fed on highly nutritious diets than on feed of a lower nutritional value. For example, it has been shown under experimental conditions that the death rate is higher in infected birds fed on a simple cereal diet to which had been added high levels of either fish meal or ground nut meal than among those receiving cereals plus much lower levels of protein supplements.

As in the case of pullorum disease, breed has an important influence on the severity of fowl typhoid, particularly where pure breeds are involved. Generally, birds of the lighter breeds, for example White Leghorns, are more resistant to the disease than heavier breeds such as Rhode Island Reds. Since the vast majority of modern layers are hybrids this effect is probably not of much significance under practical conditions.

Finally, there is the influence of age on the severity of infection and, in this respect, fowl typhoid differs markedly from all other salmonella infections of poultry, including pullorum disease and *Salmonella typhi-murium* and *thompson* infections, these diseases producing severe effects only in young chicks and growers, adults, in general, being highly resistant to fatal infection. Fowl typhoid, however, is severe in both chicks and adults.

Post Mortem Findings

In birds that die within six to eight days of exhibiting signs of ill health, that is during the acute phase of the disease, the changes in the internal organs are fairly constant, but they are not sufficiently characteristic to establish a definite diagnosis of fowl typhoid. This can be achieved only as a result of a laboratory examination. The liver and spleen are almost invariably found to be enlarged and, in some cases, the liver has a rather typical greenish-bronze colour. The intestines are severely inflamed and contain a greenish-yellow slimy fluid. The flesh is usually congested and feverish-looking,

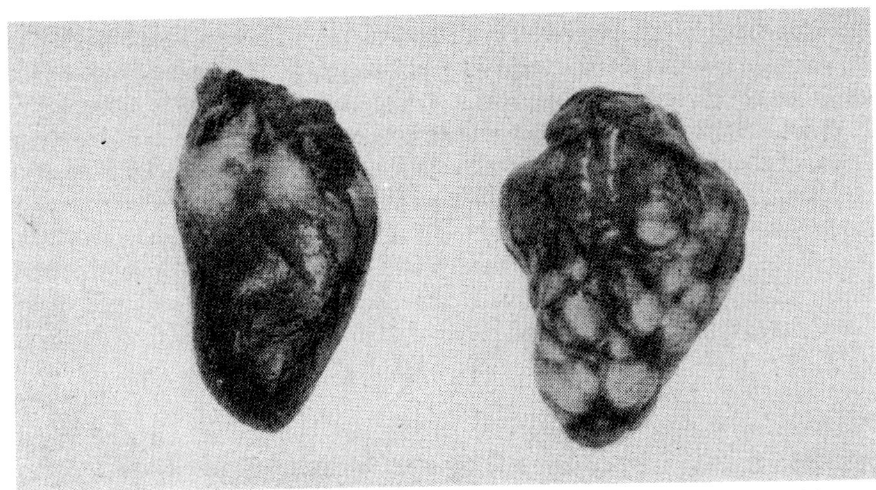

3.1   Heart from a long standing case of fowl typhoid (right) and normal heart. Note the large greyish-white nodules bulging out from the surface of the diseased heart.

but there is little wasting of the muscles.

By contrast, wasting is very pronounced in birds that die during the chronic phase of the disease, the carcase consisting of little more than skin and bone. Large greyish white nodules may bulge out from the surface of the heart of birds that have died from the chronic disease. Similar nodules which occasionally break down to form into ulcers may be found at post-mortem examination to be scattered throughout the intestine. Much smaller greyish white areas, little more than of pin-head size, may be observed on the surface of the liver.

Diagnosis

Signs and post mortem changes should give rise to suspicion of the disease and this is confirmed by isolation of the organism in the laboratory. Isolation is best achieved from the livers and spleens of freshly dead birds. There may be some difficulty in distinguishing between *Salmonella gallinarum* and *Salmonella pullorum*, but since most cases occur in adult birds, and pollorum disease only affects chicks this in itself should serve as a distinguishing factor.

Source of Outbreaks

Birds that recover from fowl typhoid continue to eliminate *Salmonella gallinarum* in their droppings and if food or water contaminated with this material is consumed by susceptible birds they will develop the disease. After being swallowed, the bacteria pass through the intestinal wall, enter the blood stream and thus set up the typical disease.

During the acute phase, affected subjects eliminate very large numbers of *Salmonella gallinarum* bacteria in their droppings and, if the conditions are right, this may soon infect others, when a typical outbreak may be set up. Elimination of the *Salmonella gallinarum* bacteria in the droppings may continue for 80 days or more *after* contracting the disease.

After infected droppings are voided the *Salmonella gallinarum* they contain can remain alive for six weeks or longer depending on the environmental conditions. For example, they have been shown to live longer in droppings that become dry after they are voided by infected birds than in those that remain moist.

Apart from infecting the droppings, *Salmonella gallinarum* may become localised in the ovaries of infected female birds in the same way as occurs in the case of *Salmonella pullorum*. Up to 50 per cent of birds that contract the disease may lay infected eggs for long periods afterwards, up to two years. With regard to the proportion of infected eggs laid by these birds, *Salmonella gallinarum* has been found in 108 of 1,843 eggs laid by 21 recovered birds. These infected eggs are liable to give rise to outbreaks in chicks if they are used for hatching. American workers have reported outbreaks in adult birds through these birds eating eggs laid by birds that had suffered from the disease. The carcases of birds that have died from fowl typhoid may also give rise to fresh outbreaks if they are not properly disposed of.

Purchased carrier birds are a common method whereby infection is introduced to a clean farm. It may also be transmitted by contaminated crates, vehicles, equipment and the clothing and boots of attendants. Once the disease is introduced to a farm it often establishes itself there and recurs from year to year unless strenuous efforts are made to eradicate it. For example of thirty—nine farms in Yorkshire which had fowl typhoid in 1952, outbreaks recurred on seventeen of them in 1953.

Finally the possibility of wild birds carrying fowl typhoid from farm to farm may be mentioned. *Salmonella gallinarum* was found in seven rooks and one pigeon in areas of Yorkshire in which fowl typhoid was common. By contrast it was not found in any of thirty-seven rooks from other parts of the country where the disease was uncommon.

PREVENTION AND CONTROL

As in the case of pullorum disease and other Salmonella infections of chicks, the drugs *furazolidone* and *furaltadone* are highly effective in treatment. As soon as a diagnosis is confirmed, surviving birds should be fed on mash containing 0.04 per cent furazolidone for ten days, or furazolidone or furaltadone given in the drinking water. Furaltadone is generally preferred as it is more soluble than furazolidone. They should then be moved to clean premises and given a further 10 day course of treatment. This is designed to prevent an outbreak after the end of the first dosage in birds that did not contract the disease initially. These birds would not have developed an immunity and would therefore be fully susceptible to infection. Such a risk does not apply in pullorum disease and the other Salmonella infections of chicks because by the time batches of chicks have completed their first course of furazolidone they have reached an age at which they are resistant. The infected premises should be thoroughly cleaned and disinfected and the buildings fumigated. Strict hygiene measures should then be taken to prevent infection being mechanically re-transmitted to the clean premises.

Another method of control is to vaccinate all birds in an affected flock a few days after completing a ten day course of furazolidone. A vaccine known as "9R" was at one time used in Britain but is not now permitted or indeed required in this country. In countries where the disease is still a problem, however, the vaccine may be used and is reasonably effective. It may also be used to prevent the disease on clean premises. The best age for vaccination is eight to fifteen weeks. At this age vaccination produces no check to growth and by the time the birds reach the period of greatest susceptibility, i.e., when they come into lay, they have developed a satisfactory immunity. One disadvantage of the vaccine is that it needs to be injected so that all birds must be handled.

One of the most important methods of control of fowl typhoid is the removal of carriers from breeding flocks by means of blood testing as in pullorum disease. The same materials and methods are used in testing for each disease and the procedure results in the elimination of reactors to both diseases. Prevention of egg transmission of the disease is achieved by this means and this goes a long way towards preventing introduction of infection to clean premises. Rigorous application of this and other control methods in Britain has almost eliminated the disease from this country. It is in less advanced countries where infection of breeding flocks is not adequately controlled that the disease persists. Chicks should be purchased only from flocks which have been blood tested and found to be 100 per cent negative to both pullorum disease and fowl typhoid.

Prevention of egg transmission will not, of course, result in overnight eradication of the disease from a country as other reservoirs of infection will persist, but it is certainly a significant step on the road to freedom from the disease.

CHAPTER 4

Avian Salmonellosis

NATURE OF DISEASE

Salmonellae are one of the most important groups of bacteria responsible for disease in poultry and other animals, including man. They comprise a large group of over a thousand serotypes some of which may infect several species of animals, whereas others infect only one or two, producing specific, well defined diseases. A good example of the latter is typhoid in man, caused by *Salmonella typhi*, an organism which infects no other species except man.

In poultry, Salmonellae produce two specific diseases; pullorum disease and fowl typhoid, caused by *Salmonella pullorum* and *Salmonella gallinarum* respectively. A great many other types of Salmonellae infect poultry and these are generally grouped together and referred to as Salmonellosis or paratyphoid. Hence the term Salmonellosis in poultry refers to infection by any Salmonella **except** *S.pullorum* or *S. gallinarum*. It is this disease with which the present chapter is concerned; pullorum disease and fowl typhoid are considered elsewhere. Although many different Salmonellae can infect poultry from time to time, one or two particular species, e.g., *Salmonella typhimurium*, occur more frequently than others and account for the majority of outbreaks.

The importance of Salmonellosis lies not only in its economic effects on the poultry industry, although these may be considerable, but also in its disease causing potential in the human population, in which Salmonellae are one of the prime causes of food poisoning. Many cases of food poisoning have been shown to have their origin in infected poultry meat and it is this association between poultry meat and Salmonellosis which has made the disease

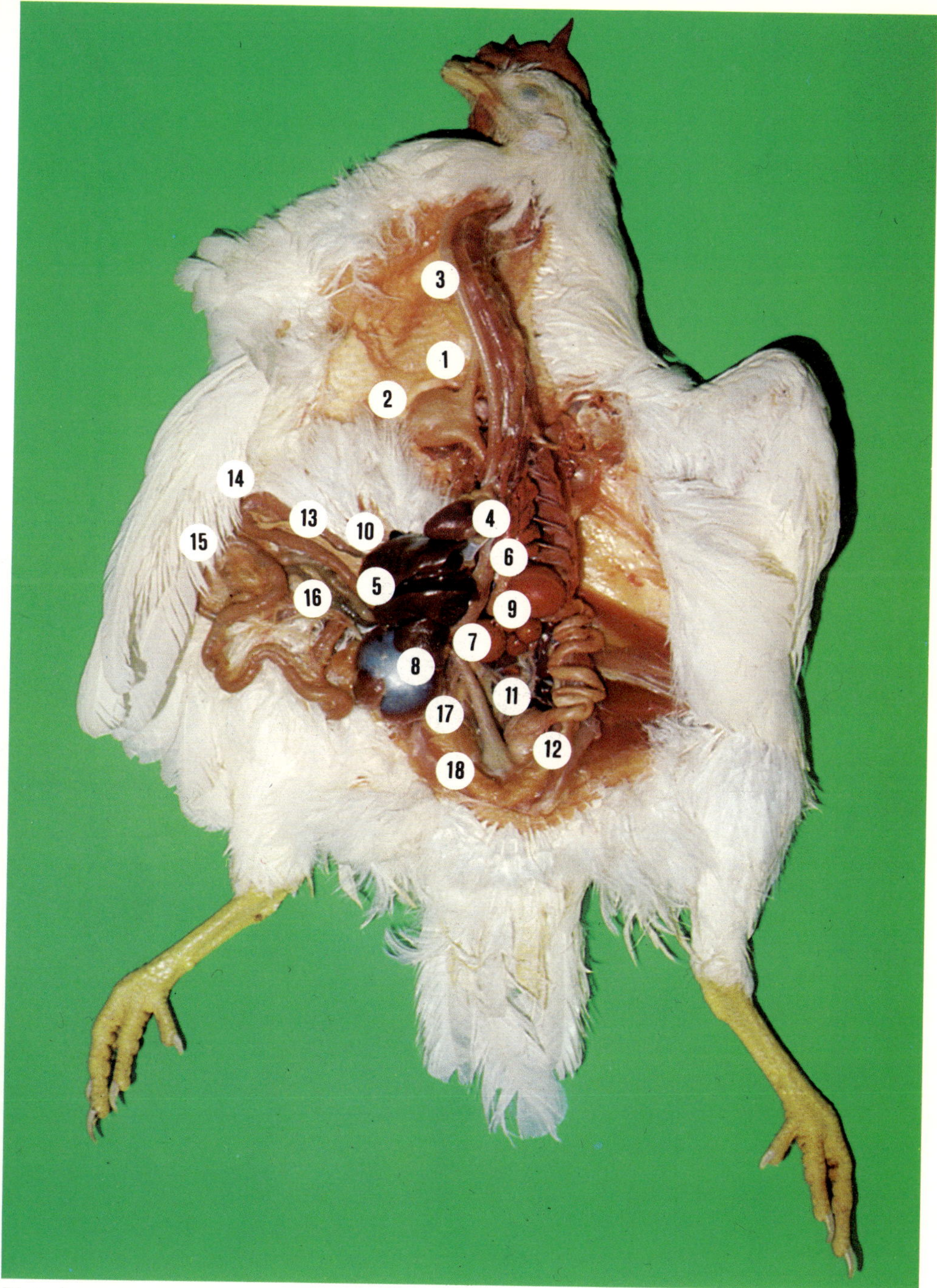

Plate 1

1 Oesophagus; 2 Crop; 3 Trachea; 4 Heart; 5 Liver; 6 Lung; 7 Proventriculus; 8 Gizzard; 9 Ovary; 10 Spleen; 11 Kidneys; 12 Oviduct; 13 Pancreas; 14 Duodenal loop; 15 Small intestine; 16 Caeca; 17 Large intestine; 18 Cloaca

Reproduced by kind permission of Intervet International, Boxmeer, The Netherlands.

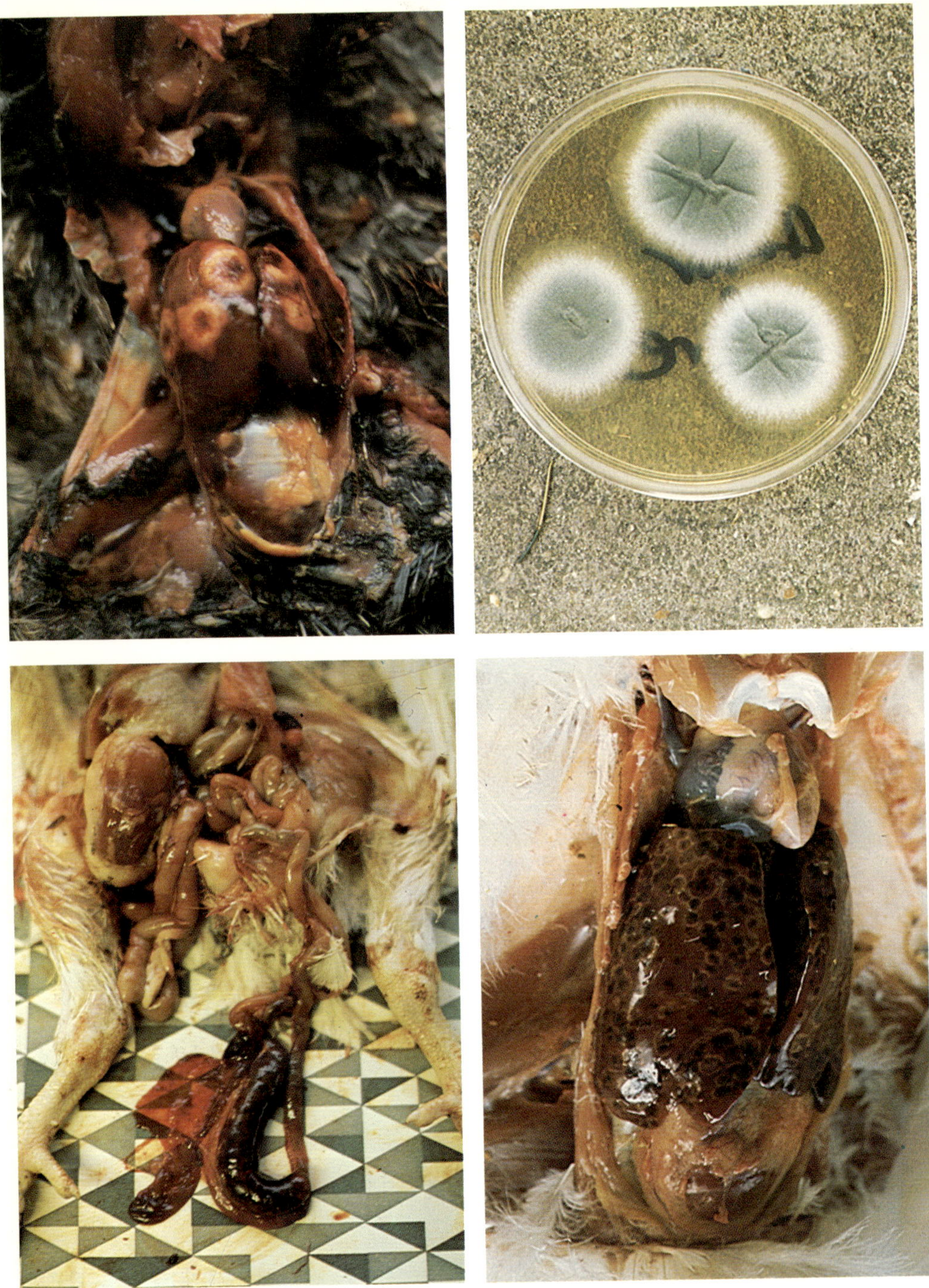

Plate 2

Upper Left: Avian Tuberculosis. Tubercular Lesions in liver of pheasant.

Upper Right: Aspergills fumigatus growing on Sabouraud's medium in the laboratory.

Lower Left: Caecal coccidiosis. Four week old chick showing severe haemorrhage in the caecal tubes, one of which has been opened.

Lower Right: Blackhead. Typical circular lesions in turkey liver.

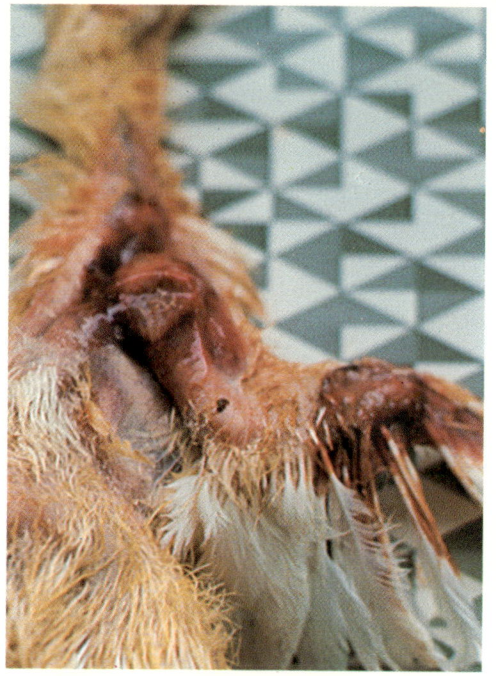

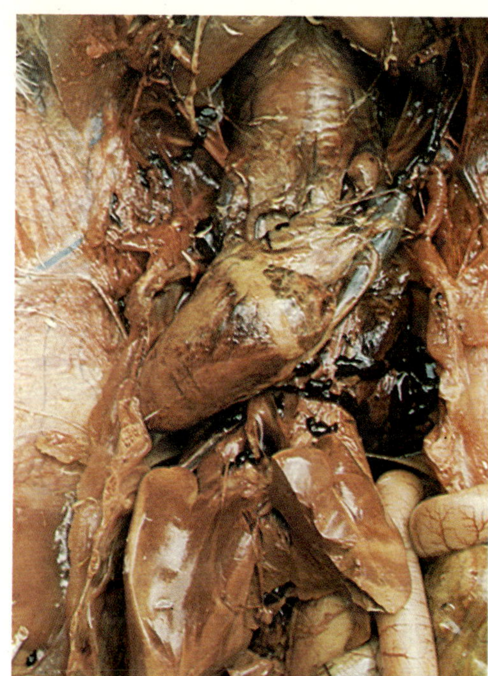

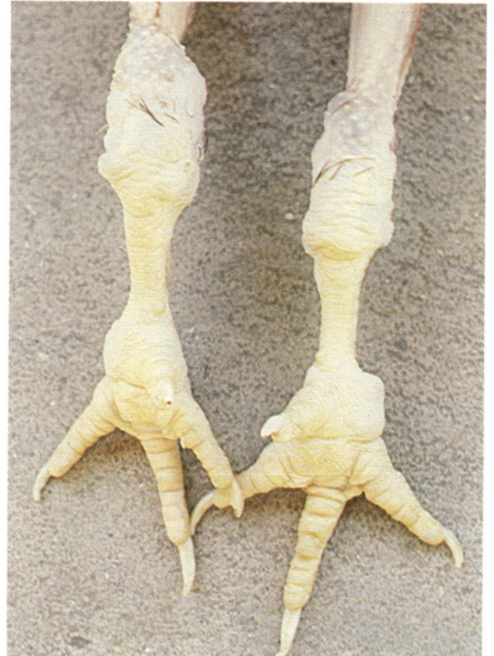

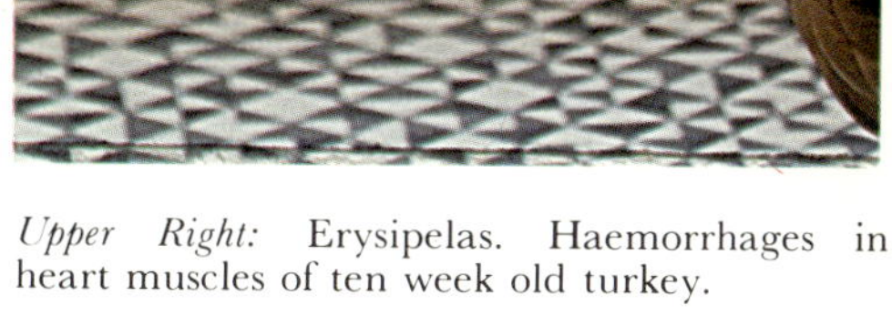

Plate 3

Upper Left: Gangrenous dermatitis. The condition is sometimes called "Wing-rot" for reasons which will be apparent from the photograph.

Lower Left: Infectious synovitis. Swelling of feet and hock joints due to *Mycoplasma synoviae* infection.

Upper Right: Erysipelas. Haemorrhages in heart muscles of ten week old turkey.

Lower Right: Swollen facial sinuses due to *Mycoplasma gallisepticum* infection. Although this photograph shows a hen, the condition is more typically seen in turkeys.

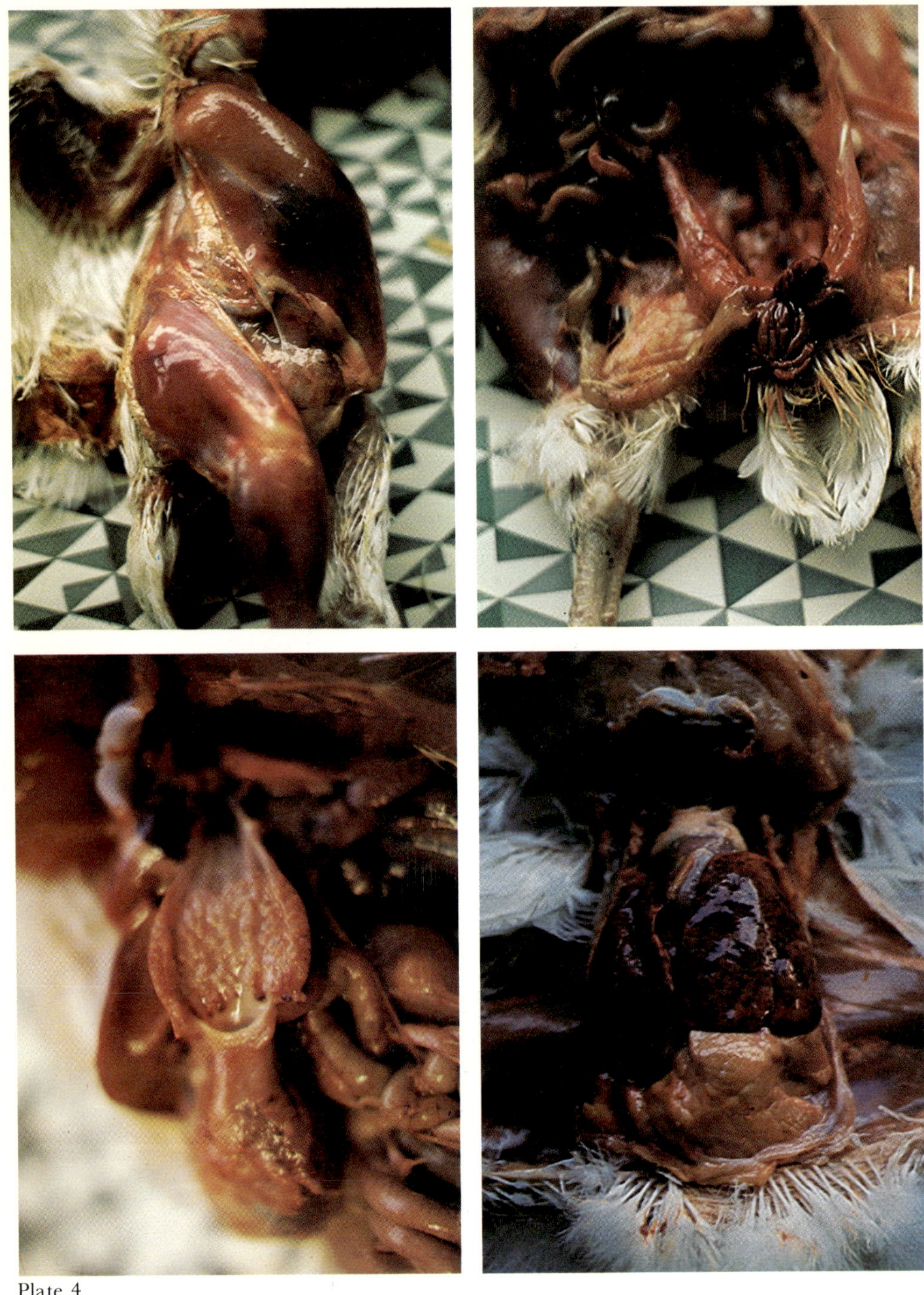

Plate 4

Upper Left: ·Infectious bursal disease. Haemorrhages in breast and thigh muscles of five week old broiler.

Upper Right: Infectious bursal disease. Inflammation of cloacal bursa.

Lower Left: Infectious bursal disease. Haemorrhages in mucous membrane of proventriculus at its junction with the gizzard.

Lower right: Inclusion – body hepatitis. Haemorrhages over liver surface in six week old broiler.

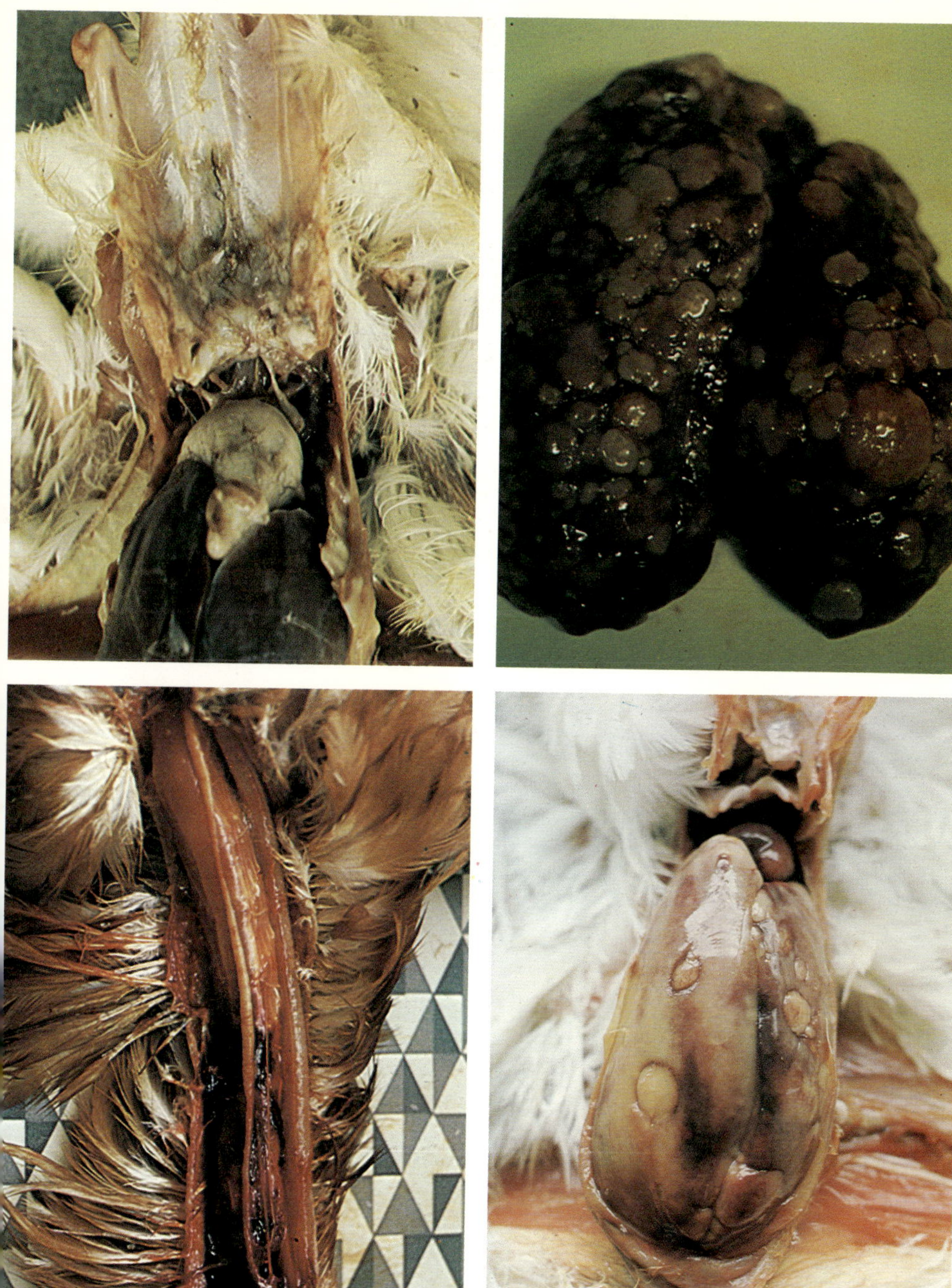

Plate 5

Upper Left: Colisepticaemia in six week old broiler. Note white fibrinous deposit over heart and liver.

Upper Right: Marek's disease. Nodular lesions in liver.

Lower Left: Marek's disease. Enlargement of vagus nerve in neck. The varying thickness of the nerve along its length can be appreciated.

Lower Right: Lymphoid leucosis. Gross swelling and paleness of liver which fills almost the entire abdomen.

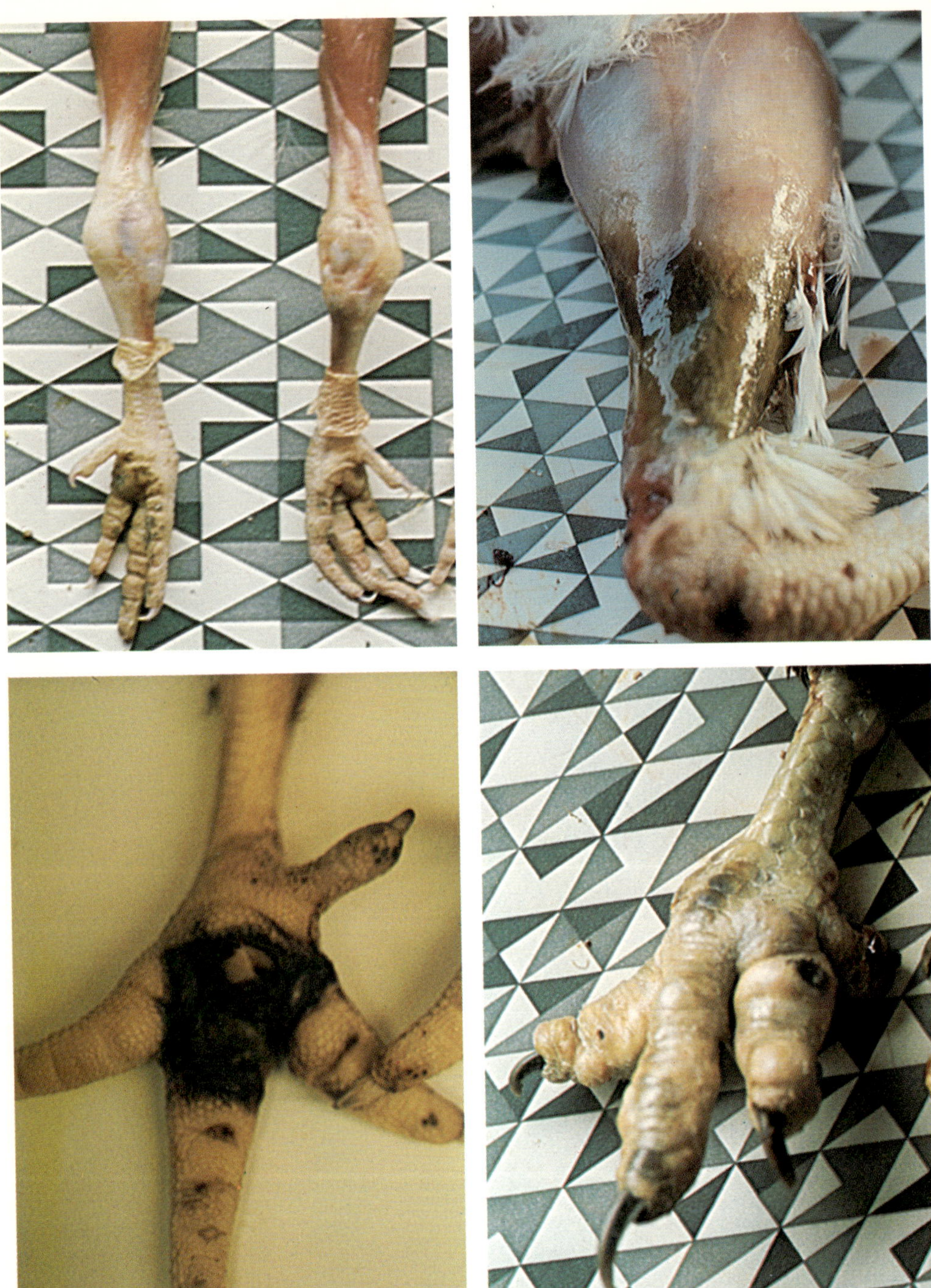

Plate 6

Upper Left: Slipped tendon. In the leg on the right the gastrocnemius tendon has slipped from its normal position on the point of the hock. In the other leg the tendon occupies its correct position.

Lower Left: Ulceration of the undersides of the feet in a bird which was kept in a small unhygienic run in a period of wet weather. (Plantar pododermatitis).

Upper Right: Ruptured tendon. The skin has been removed to show green discolouration of the underlying tissues which frequently occurs following rupture or tearing of the gastrocnemius tendon above the hock.

Lower Right: Articular gout. Swelling of the feet due to deposition of urates in and around joints following kidney damage.

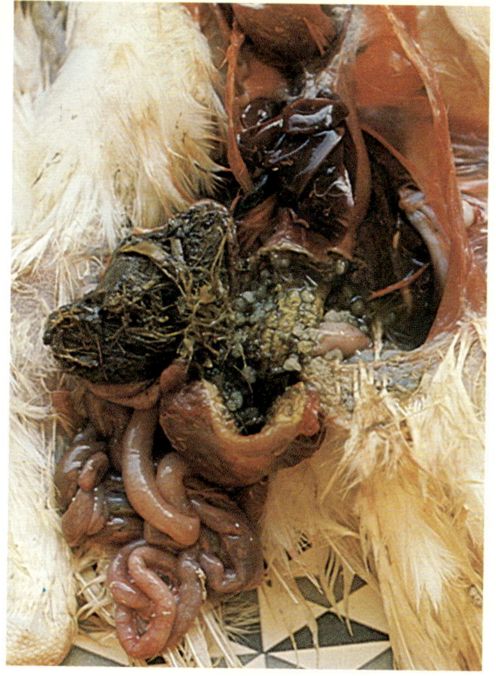

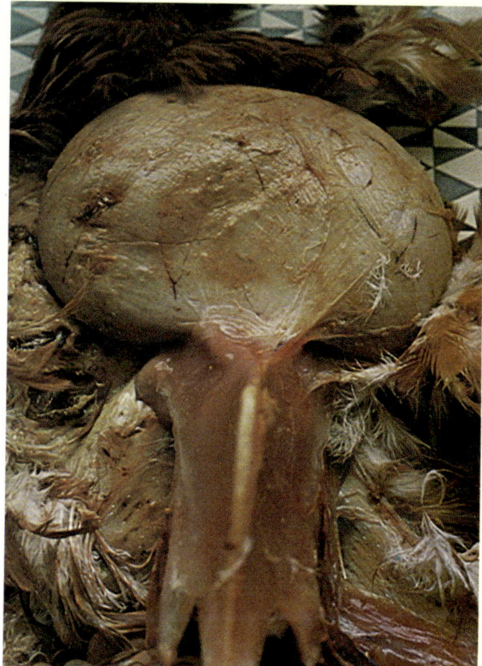

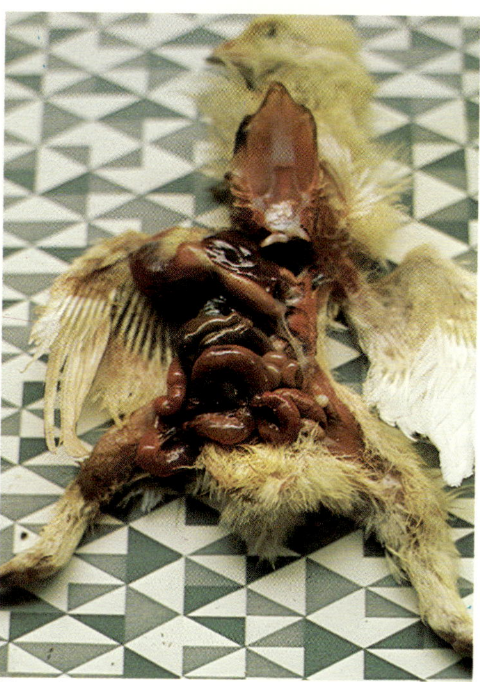

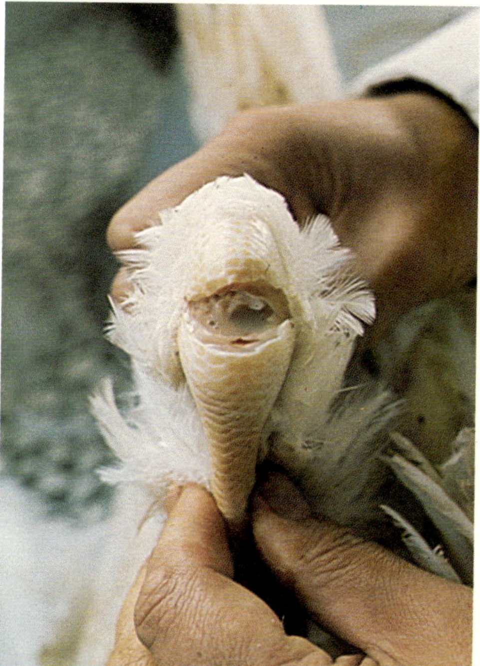

Plate 7

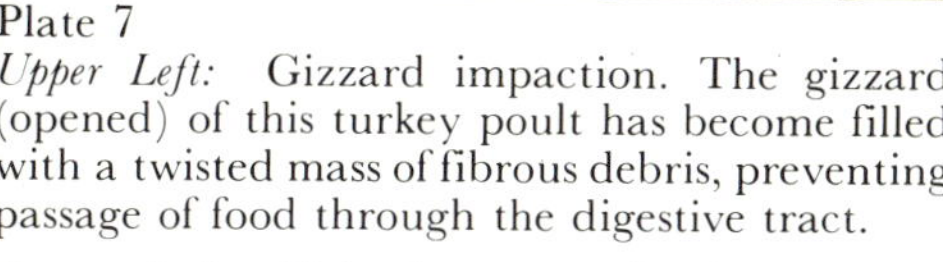

Upper Left: Gizzard impaction. The gizzard (opened) of this turkey poult has become filled with a twisted mass of fibrous debris, preventing passage of food through the digestive tract.

Lower Left: Volvulus or twisted gut. The intestines have become twisted on themselves causing obstruction. The affected loops of bowel are severaly inflamed. The condition should not be confused with coccidiosis.

Upper Right: Sour crop. The crop is greatly enlarged and filled with sour smelling food material. Note the resulting poor condition of the bird.

Lower Right: Staphylococcal arthritis. The hock joint has been opened to show the white, purulent fluid in the joint.

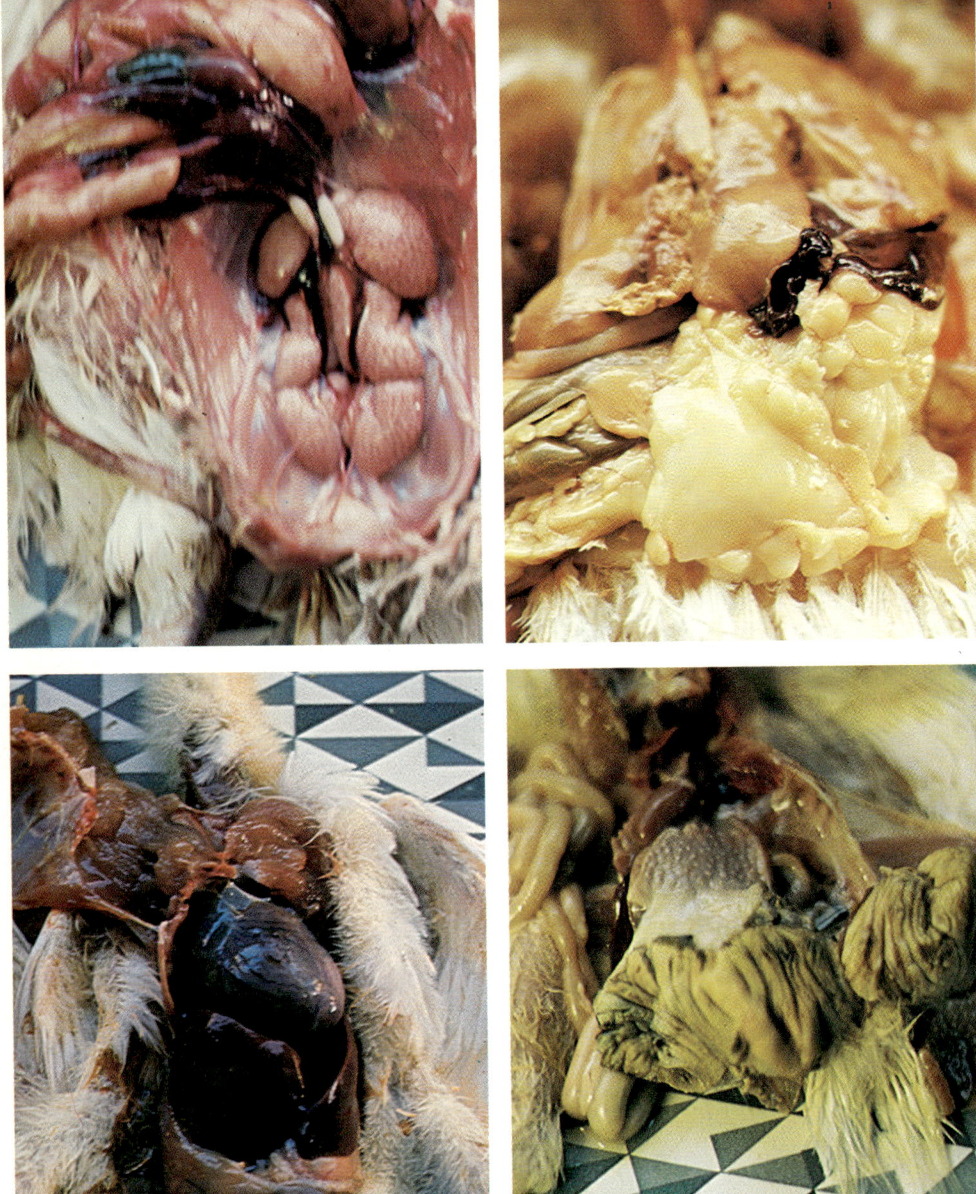

Plate 8

Upper Left: Swelling and pallor kidneys. The cause of this type of kidney damage is uncertain but it is believed in some cases to be associated with infectious bronchitis virus infection.

Lower Left: Round heart disease in the turkey poult. The heart is enlarged and the rounded shape can be appreciated.

Upper Right: Fatty liver haemorrhagic syndrome. The liver is pale and soft due to fatty infiltration. There is excess abdominal fat and a large blood clot lies under the liver, having resulted from its rupture.

Lower Right: Gizzard erosion in the broiler. The gizzard has been opened to show dark coloured erosions and ulcers.

the subject of much discussion and at times emotive debate among members of the farming community, the food industry, the health authorities, the veterinary and medical professions and other interested parties. Salmonellosis indeed is now a notifiable disease under the Zoonosis order and steps have been taken to control it, with some success. Eradication of the disease however is still a long way in the future, if ever it becomes possible.

CAUSE

As stated, the cause of Salmonellosis is infection by any species of Salmonella except *Salmonella pullorum* and *Salmonella gallinarum*. Some of the commoner types found in poultry are *Salmonella typhimurium, Salmonella inf.. tis, Salmonella enteritidis* and *Salmonella thompson*. Many other types are isolated only on rare occasions from single flocks or single birds and generally cause no disease or only low mortality.

OCCURRENCE

Salmonellosis occurs in all types of poultry on a world wide scale. In countries with a progressive poultry industry it has been controlled to a large extent by improved hygiene methods on breeding farms and in hatcheries. It should be said, however, that although clinical disease has been largely controlled, infection rates in the poultry population may be higher than the number of disease outbreaks would indicate. Isolations of Salmonellae are still made not infrequently from broiler or turkey flocks or litter and poultry slaughter plants. Certainly Salmonellae are widespread in nature and the possibility of their gaining entry to poultry flocks is ever present. In the majority of cases of infection no clinical disease results, the importance of the infection being the possibility that pathogenic Salmonellae may be transmitted to the human population.

Salmonellosis still poses a considerable threat to the poultry industries of developing countries, in which hygiene standards may be less than optimal and in which outbreaks may still be relatively frequent. It sometimes happens that a particular Salmonella type is isolated in an area and then, apparently by spreading to other flocks, becomes common in that area, later becoming endemic or again decreasing in incidence. Certain types may be relatively common in one country and much rarer in another. New serotypes continue to be isolated but many of the exotic types cause little or no disease whereas the more prevalent types such as *typhimurium* tend to be highly pathogenic.

SPREAD

Salmonella organisms are harboured in the intestines and gall bladder of symptomless carrier birds and are passed in the faeces. These organisms may contaminate egg-shells as eggs are laid, or through the medium of dirty nest boxes or floors of breeding houses. Egg shell contamination in the hatchery may also occur. The organisms are capable of penetrating the shell, particularly during cooling of the egg, or if eggs   washed, multiplying within the egg and causing Salmonellosis in the hatched chick. **This is the main method of transmission of the disease;** true ovarian transmission in the chicken is a relatively rare occurence although it may occur not uncommonly in the turkey and rather frequently in the duck. After hatching, the chick, poult or duckling can then pass the infection to its hatch mates, either on the hatcher trays or in the brooder house, very few infected chicks being necessary to give rise to a major outbreak of disease.

Spread of Salmonellosis can also occur in other ways. Various animal species, particularly rodents may act as a source of infection and spread the disease to poultry by contaminating food, water or litter. Infection can also be spread by the use of contaminated equipment and on attendants' hands, boots, etc., especially if one person is looking after both young chicks and older birds in which carriers may exist.

It is now well recognised that various exotic Salmonella serotypes can be introduced to poultry via feed which contains infected protein of animal origin, e.g., meat and bone meal or fish meal. This in fact is now considered to be one of the main sources of infection of broiler flocks. It has been shown that where contaminated food is supplied to a breeding flock, the flock may acquire the infection, which can then survive the entire chain of broiler production, i.e., fertile egg, hatchery, broiler flock, processing plant and retailer, with the possibility of a food poisoning outbreak in the consumer.

In any discussion of Salmonellosis the danger of infection of the human population must be considered. In the case of poultry this may occur through the medium of infected poultry meat or infected eggs or egg products. When infected birds enter a poultry killing plant, dissemination of infection is likely to occur in spite of rigorous hygiene standards being applied within the plant. Dissemination is apparently most likely to occur in the scald tank and plucking machines, but may also occur at other points. The introduction of the *Poultry Meat (Hygiene) Regulations (1976)* with improved structural and hygiene standards in killing plants should significantly reduce dissemination of bacterial organisms and cross-contamination of carcases in killing plants.

Salmonella organisms may be preserved in infected carcases by freezing and may not be killed by cooking if the temperature or time of cooking are incorrect. *The importance of correct thawing and cooking procedures cannot be over-emphasised.* Thus the final defence against Salmonella food poisoning derived from poultry rests with the housewife or other persons who may be involved with cooking poultry meat; adequate cooking will destroy any organisms which have survived all other stages of the production chain.

Food poisoning outbreaks have also resulted from contamination of liquid or dried egg or egg products. Since the introduction of pasteurisation regulations for liquid egg, however, outbreaks from this source have been almost totally eliminated.

Signs

Signs of Salmonellosis **in poultry** are almost totally confined to young chicks, poults or ducklings under three weeks of age. Although older birds may be carriers of infection, they themselves rarely show any evidence of disease.

In young birds signs include drowsiness, closed eyes, ruffled feathers and a desire for heat. There may be severe diarrhoea and vent pasting. Affected chicks lose their appetite but may show increased thirst.

Generally when Salmonellosis occurs **in chicks** of less than one week of age the source of infection is likely to be the hatchery or the hatching egg. If first signs of the disease are seen in birds older than one week an external source of infection such as food is likely. Mortality in either case may be 50 per cent of the flock or more, the severity of an outbreak depending on the type of organism involved, the general health of the chicks and the standard of management.

In Salmonellosis **in ducklings** sudden death immediately after drinking may be a prominent feature.

In rare cases of clinical Salmonellosis **in older birds** there is acute disease of short duration with thirst, inappetance, diarrhoea and general malaise. Recovery is generally rapid and mortality low.

Post Mortem Findings

Post mortem findings in Salmonellosis are neither constant nor characteristic. They may depend to some degree on the species of Salmonella involved. In *typhimurium* infection in young chicks however, the most common changes are enlargement of the liver, with necrotic foci and sometimes haemorrhages scattered over its surface, pericarditis, the pericardial sac being thickened, opaque and yellow-white in colour, thickening of the air sacs and caseous accumulations or "cores" in the caecal tubes. There may also be haemorrhagic enteritis, enlargement of the spleen and infection of the yolk sac.

Frequently chick carcases are emaciated and dehydrated. In extremely acute outbreaks, no visible changes may be present in many of the chicks. In adult birds changes are less distinct but generally consist of swelling of the liver, spleen and kidneys with sometimes pericarditis, peritonitis and enteritis. The reproductive tract may also be involved with degeneration of ova in the ovary and purulent or caseous accumulations in the oviduct. In some cases this oviduct involvement progresses to generalised peritonitis. In adult carrier birds no lesions are usually visible.

DIAGNOSIS

Salmonellosis cannot be diagnosed accurately from clinical signs or post mortem findings although these should give rise to suspicion of the disease. For confirmation live or freshly dead chicks should be submitted to a laboratory for isolation and identification of the causative organism. This is a relatively complex procedure and specimens should be sent to a laboratory where the necessary expertise exists for this work.

In the case of flocks in which there exist adult carriers, culture of cloacal swabs may detect infected birds. However this procedure is not as accurate as might be desired since excretion of organisms is intermittent. Culture of litter from several areas of a house is a useful procedure for detecting infected flocks although it does not, of course, detect individually infected birds.

TREATMENT

Outbreaks of Salmonellosis in young chicks are generally treated

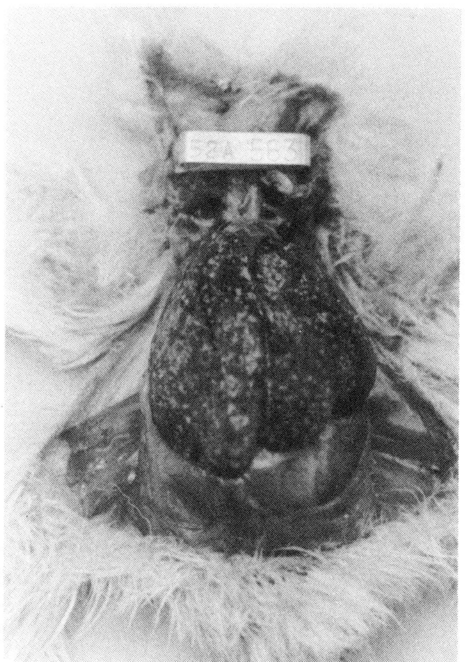

4.1   Avian Salmonellosis in week old chick. The liver is enlarged and its surface covered with pin-head sized, or slightly larger, greyish-white nodules.

with the drug **Furazolidone** in the water or the food. Where water treatment is used the closely related and more soluble compound **Furaltadone** may be used. These compounds give rapid control of an outbreak, but have the disadvantage that they do not completely eliminate infection so that many recovered birds become carriers. For this reason flocks that have been treated for Salmonellosis should not be reared for future breeding stock.

Other anti-microbial substances have been used to treat Salmonellosis in the past, but Furazolidone is so much more effective than other known drugs that these are rarely used and need not be considered further.

In the case of infected broiler flocks a course of treatment may be given before slaughter in addition to treatment in the stage of active disease. This is an attempt, on public health grounds, to reduce the numbers of Salmonella organisms carried by recovered birds and therefore the numbers of organisms entering the killing plant.

PREVENTION AND CONTROL.

It was mentioned in the chapters dealing with Pullorum disease and fowl typhoid that excellent control of these diseases has been achieved by blood testing of parent stock and elimination of reactors. Unfortunately, for a number of reasons no such test is available to detect birds infected by other types of Salmonellae. Preventive measures must therefore be directed to hygiene practices at the supply farms which produce hatching eggs, at the hatchery and in the brooding house. True ovarian transmission of Salmonellosis, in chickens at any rate, is rare, and prevention therefore depends on the production of clean eggs in which contamination of the shell is avoided.

Important procedures in this respect include keeping nest boxes clean, frequent collection of eggs, avoiding the use of floor laid eggs and correct storage and transport. Prevention of penetration of the shell by the organism will largely control the disease.

Important Procedures

1. **Eggs should be fumigated with formaldehyde immediately after collection and stored in a proper egg storage room at a temperature of 55°F (12.7°C) and relative humidity of 75 per cent.**

Egg dipping may also be used but should be carried out using correct equipment according to the manufacturer's instructions, at the correct temperature which must always be higher than that of the eggs. Wiping of egg shells with a damp cloth and cold water will result in penetration of the shell by Salmonellae or other organisms which happen to be on the shell. This procedure will thus have the opposite effect to that which is intended and should never be used. Such heavily contaminated eggs should not be used for hatching purposes.

2. **The highest standards of hygiene in the hatchery are necessary to prevent contamination of the egg shell and outbreaks of Salmonellosis, or indeed, other egg transmitted diseases.**

Eggs should be stored for as short a time as possible before setting, again under correct conditions of temperature and relative humidity, and repeat fumigation should be carried out before setting. Although it is possible to fumigate during incubation this procedure may result in damage to embryos and should on no account be carried out between the twenty-fourth and ninety-sixth hours of incubation.

3. **Incubators should be thoroughly cleaned and fumigated after each hatch and hatching trays, trolleys and other equipment disinfected.**
4. **Routine monitoring of hatchery fluff, dead-in-shell embryos and air samples to check the level of contamination is an important part of a hatchery hygiene programme.**
5. **High standards of hygiene and management at the brooding premises are also necessary to prevent Salmonella infection or minimise losses where infected chicks are delivered.**

It must be remembered that although egg transmission is the main source of infection in young chicks, infection can be introduced by other means. Hence chicks should be delivered to a house which has been thoroughly cleaned out, disinfected and fumigated; new litter should be used and rodents, and wild birds, should be excluded. The use of Furazolidone in the food as a preventive measure, while not taking the place of good hygiene and management, can be beneficial where Salmonellosis is suspected or where, for example, it is known that a previous broiler crop was infected. The ever present possibility of introduction of Salmonella organisms in the feed must also be borne in mind. In the case of broiler and turkey feed the pelleting process may reduce, but not eliminate, this source of infection.

CHAPTER 5

Avian Tuberculosis

NATURE OF DISEASE

One of the most important diseases of chickens in Britain in the earlier years of this century, **avian tuberculosis** is now rarely seen except in an occasional free-range "back-yard" flock. Part of the reason for this is that tuberculosis is a very chronic condition and since most birds are now killed at the end of their first laying year the disease has insufficient time in which to manifest itself. Over the years this has resulted in a reduced incidence of the organism in the environment and a further reduction in the number of clinical cases of tuberculosis. The disease may, however, be of major importance in certain countries whose poultry industries still consist of mainly small flocks kept under less than optimal conditions of health and hygiene. Certainly it occurred world wide before the development of the modern poultry industry. The disease affects mainly chickens, but turkeys, ducks, geese and game birds, particularly pheasants, are also susceptible.

CAUSE

Tuberculosis occurs in many animal species and is caused by a bacterial organism known properly as *Mycobacterium tuberculosis*, or, more commonly, as the *tubercle bacillus*. Several types and strains of the bacillus exist which infect primarily one species of animal. The most important strains are the **human, bovine** and **avian.** Fowls are infected by the avian strain, this strain also being commonly found in localised tuberculous lesions in pigs. Cases of infection with the avian strain have been recorded in humans, but these are extremely rare. Tubercle bacilli are very resistant to external influences and have been found to survive for at least one year in buried tuberculous carcases. They are killed by direct sunlight but not if, as is usually the case, they are protected by droppings, soil or other material.

SPREAD

Spread of the disease occurs mainly by contamination of food and water with organisms passed in very large numbers in the droppings of infected birds in which ulceration of the bowel has occurred. Spread by contaminated utensils, attendants' boots etc. is also possible and the organism may be introduced to a flock by wild birds. The longevity of the organism in contaminated ground, litter, etc., must be borne in mind when putting poultry on "clean" ground. Viable organisms may still be present in such ground although no birds have been kept on it for many months.

Course

Tuberculosis runs a prolonged, chronic course, signs of the disease seldom being seen in birds of less than one year of age. Consequently it is unknown in the broiler industry and seldom occurs in layers killed at the end of their first laying year. Because of its protracted course it is generally seen only in small, free-range flocks in which birds have been allowed to survive to an advanced age.

Mortality rate in tuberculosis is generally low, an occasional bird being lost from time to time in an affected flock.

The signs of tuberculosis are not specific, but the main sign is chronic loss of weight and condition. This may be apparent visually but it is best detected by handling the birds, when loss of flesh over the breast bone will be evident. Eventually the stage of gross emaciation is reached. Other signs which may be present are paleness and shrinking of the comb, diarrhoea and lameness when joints are affected. In some cases death may occur when the affected bird is still in relatively good condition, due to tuberculous lesions in internal organs resulting, for example, in rupture of the liver.

Appetite generally remains good until shortly before death, even in cases of extreme emaciation.

Post Mortem Findings

The lesions of tuberculosis are characteristic and easily recog-

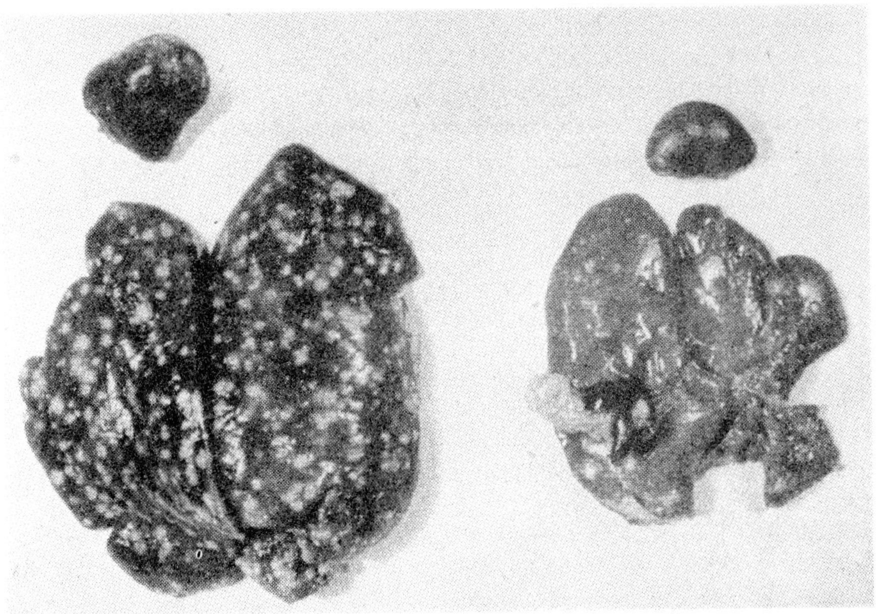

5.1 Liver and spleen of a bird suffering from tuberculosis (left) covered with greyish-white or pale yellow nodules. A healthy liver and spleen are seen on the right.

nised on post mortem. Affected carcases are usually in very poor condition. The organs most commonly affected are the liver, spleen, intestine and bone marrow. In the liver multiple, yellow-white caseous nodules are found. These vary in size from pin-head to pea or larger and they may occur singly, or fuse to form a large tubercular mass. The lesions in the spleen are similar but are often larger and tend to protrude from the surface of the organ giving it an irregular shape.

The liver and spleen may be normal in size but are usually enlarged to some degree. Ocasionally a blood clot is found in the abdominal cavity due to rupture of one of these organs.

Nodular lesions are also found in the walls of the intestines. Some of these lesions give rise to ulceration of the interior of the intestine from which very large numbers of organisms escape into the intestinal lumen and are passed in the droppings. Nodules are also often found in the bone marrow and in the leg joints.

Diagnosis

Diagnosis on post mortem examination is not usually difficult.

Tuberculosis should be suspected from the characteristic lesions. Confirmation is achieved by microscopic examination of material from lesions, stained by a method known as Ziehl-Neelsen. Tuberculosis is the only disease of chickens in which "acid-fast" organisms are visible microscopically when stained by this method.

Diagnosis in the live bird is possible by use of the tuberculin test. The test is not one hundred per cent accurate but gives a good indication of the presence of the disease in a flock and is especially useful in detecting early cases.

The test consists of injecting avian tuberculin into the skin of one wattle of each bird in the flock. The same wattle, either right or left, should be used in each bird and the wattles handled carefully to avoid injury which might give confusing results. The test is read in forty-eight hours and a positive reaction consists of a hot swelling of the injected wattle. The degree of swelling varies, reaching up to twice the size of the other wattle. All reacting birds should be culled. A lack of lesions in some birds giving a positive reaction may indicate early infection. Healthy birds generally give no reaction.

PREVENTION AND CONTROL

There is no treatment for affected birds, which should be culled and disposed of by burning or burying.
The tuberculin test will detect most affected birds in a flock. When these have been removed the healthy birds must be moved to clean ground to avoid their picking up infection from the soil. Further cases may occur in the healthy birds later, however, and retesting should be repeated at three monthly intervals until no further cases are detected. Moving to fresh ground each time is necessary. Clearly, this may give rise to a good deal of difficulty and except in the case of very valuable flocks, it may be easier and more economical to cull the entire flock and restock with clean birds on fresh ground.

Ground contaminated with tuberculosis organisms should be limed or ploughed and left free of poultry for at least one year. All equipment must be cleaned and disinfected and left free of use for several weeks if possible. Even when all these measures are adopted however, the total elimination of tuberculosis from an infected premises may not be easily achieved.

CHAPTER 6

Yolk Sac Infection

NATURE OF DISEASE

Yolk sac infection is a condition commonly seen in chicks and turkey poults and also in goslings and ducklings in the first week of life. The condition is one in which bacteria gain access, either before or soon after hatching, to the yolk sac which becomes absorbed into the chick's body shortly before hatching. These bacteria multiply profusely within the yolk, following which they invade the blood stream causing a generalised bacterial toxaemia and death of the chick.

Yolk sac infection is sometimes referred to as **mushy chick disease;** if the infection originated through an unhealed navel it is termed **omphalitis**. It should be made clear that many cases of yolk sac infection occur with no evidence of unhealed navels and some authorities regard yolk sac infection and omphalitis as distinct and separate conditions. Frequently however the two conditions occur together, infection gaining entry to the yolk through the navel.

Yolk sac infection is undoubtedly one of the commonest causes of loss of chicks and poults in the first few days of life. Various studies have shown that between 30 and 50 per cent of chick mortality in the first ten days of life has been due to this condition. While the incidence of the condition has fallen somewhat in recent years, due no doubt to better understanding of the underlying causes, so that appropriate preventive measures are taken, it is still a cause of serious economic loss to the industry.

In some cases death of the embryo occurs before hatching, giving an increase in the numbers of "dead-in-shell". It may be anticipated that this will be followed by a yolk sac infection problem when the chicks are placed. When a significant increase in dead-in-shell occurs the cause should always be investigated so that where possible appropriate measures can be taken to minimise losses in the hatched chicks.

SOURCE OF OUTBREAKS

When yolk sac infection first became a problem shortly after the introduction of mammoth incubators it was commonly believed that the main causes were lack of hygiene in the incubator, faulty incubation technique and failure of rapid healing of chicks' navels so that infection gained entry through the navel. Later however it was found that the condition still occurred when these faults were corrected and that other factors were involved. The most important of these was found to be bacterial contamination of the egg shell either before setting or during the period of incubation. Bacteria were found to have the ability to penetrate the egg shell and this penetration occurred most readily during the period of egg cooling when contraction of contents took place, bacteria being drawn through the shell pores. Obviously incubation of dirty eggs will greatly increase the chances of a yolk sac infection problem occurring after hatching.

Bacterial penetration of egg shells may occur if eggs are contaminated by faeces and if nest boxes are allowed to become dirty. Also floor-laid eggs are likely to be contaminated, with the possibility of a subsequent yolk sac infection problem. Unhygienic conditions of egg storage and incubation will also contribute to the problem and high humidity in the incubator will encourage bacterial growth. In addition shell penetration may occur when eggs are transferred from incubator to hatcher mainly because cooling occurs at this time and bacteria present on the shell surface can be drawn into the egg.

Yolk sac infection is not normally regarded as a contagious condition, i.e., it is not transmitted from chick to chick. However the bacterial species which cause the condition tend to be extremely common wherever chickens are raised. Many are normal inhabitants of the chickens intestinal tract as well as its environment. It is not possible to eliminate these bacterial species by blood testing as in the case of Pullorum disease, or by any other method. Pathogenic strains of these organisms are readily transmitted from chick to chick via the intestinal or respiratory routes and if the chicks become weakened through chilling or other stress, organisms may invade the yolk sac from within the chick. Such an infection is sometimes regarded as secondary, as distinct from a primary infection when penetration of the egg shell occurs.

Hence in yolk sac infections bacterial invasion can occur by three main routes:

1. penetration of the egg shell
2. through unhealed navels
3. invasion from the intestinal or respiratory tracts

The first of these is the most important route of infection.

When the causative bacteria reach the yolk they multiply profusely and produce toxic waste products which are absorbed into the blood-stream of the chick and cause its death. If this occurs early in incubation the embryo may die and will be classified as dead-in-shell. If shell penetration occurs later, or if bacterial multiplication is less rapid the chick may hatch only to die a few days later and be recorded as a victim of yolk sac infection.

A number of bacterial species can cause yolk sac infection. These include *Bacillus cereus*, *Proteus*, *Salmonella*, *Clostridia*, *Streptococci* and *Staphylococci*. The organism involved in most cases however is *Escherichia coli*. The ability of an organism to cause yolk sac infection depends on its ability to degrade or break down yolk protein. *Bacillus cereus* appears to have this property and it is thought that in many cases this organism invades first and is followed by other organisms such as *E.coli* which then find ideal growth conditions in the altered yolk, multiply rapidly and cause the death of the chick.

Signs

Signs of yolk sac infection are not characteristic and do not serve to distinguish it from other diseases of baby chicks. Affected chicks may be small and weak or they may be large and excessively moist, "mushy chicks". They usually appear unwell, lack vitality and look dejected. They may stand motionless for long periods, often with closed eyes and chirping loudly. Their appetite is poor or absent and a white diarrhoea may be present which soils the vent and gives rise to "vent-pasting". Such chicks rapidly weaken and die.

The greatest number of deaths from yolk sac infection occur in the first five days after hatching, but losses may continue up to the tenth day. The extent of the losses varies greatly from batch to batch, sometimes only a very few chicks dying. The average among affected batches is probably in the region of 2 to 5 per cent. Losses over 10 per cent are seldom experienced.

Post Mortem Findings

Chicks which have died due to yolk sac infection may be small and emaciated or they may be apparently quite large due to excessive moisture of the carcase. In any case a notable feature is usually swelling of the abdomen due to gross enlargement of the contained yolk sac. This can often be appreciated with the carcase still intact. On removing the skin the carcase musculature is often poorly developed and emaciated and the muscular tissue has a reddened, inflamed appearance. The yolk sac is enlarged with inflamed walls, the blood vessels being dilated and standing out clearly from the surrounding tissue. The yolk is usually markedly altered in appearance from the normal greenish-yellow colour and rather viscous consistency. The colour varies from dark brown to bright yellow and the consistency becomes watery with large flakes of granular, curdled material. In some cases the yolk material becomes almost completely solid. Usually it has an unpleasant smell. The precise appearance of the yolk depends on the bacterial types involved and the duration of the infection. If the infection gains entry through the navel, there will be imperfect healing of the navel and inflammation in that region.

In many cases of infected yolk sacs the infection spreads to involve other abdominal organs giving rise to a generalised peritonitis, and in those chicks which survive for several days there may also be pericarditis.

It should be noted that some bacteria can produce infection of the yolk sac without causing marked alterations in the visible appearance of the yolk. Laboratory examination is therefore necessary in those cases in which yolk sac infection is suspected, but in which yolk changes are not evident. These cases however are very much in the minority.

Diagnosis

Diagnosis of yolk sac infection is usually readily made from post mortem findings. In many cases the disease can be suspected even before death by the swollen abdomens evident in a number of chicks in the flock. Bacteriological examination of yolk sac contents will determine the bacterial organism involved in the disease in any particular case.

Treatment

Drugs, including antibiotics, are of limited value in the treatment of yolk sac infection because, although they are absorbed into the

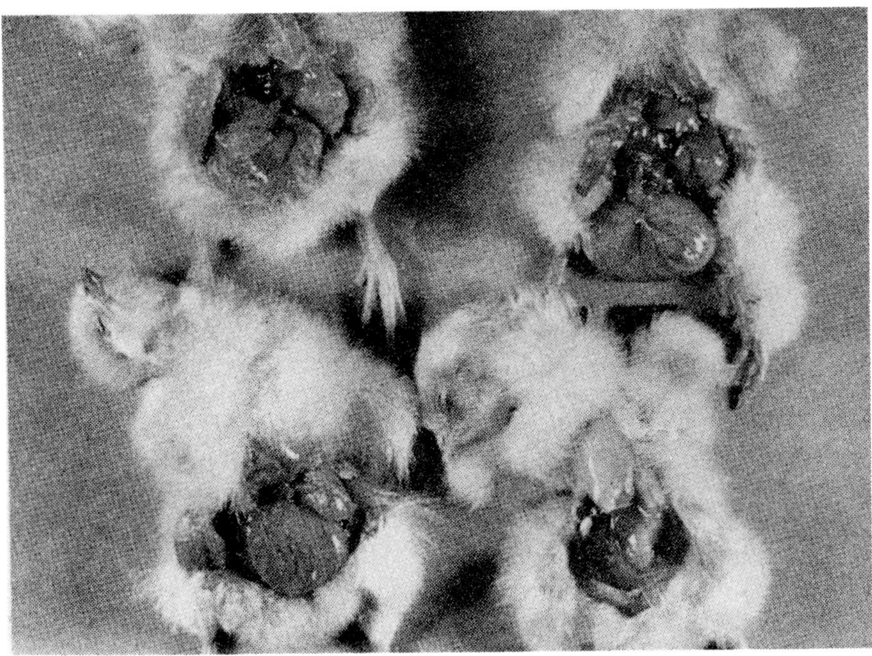

6.1 Examples of infected yolk sacs compared with the normal sac seen top left. The infected sacs are enlarged, the blood vessels being dilated and standing out clearly from the surrounding tissue.

chick's body, they do not achieve high concentration in the yolk, the seat of infection. However, they may help to prevent further cases developing and have some beneficial effect on the health of the flock as a whole, and many cases of yolk sac infection are treated with antibacterial substances such as the tetracyclines and furazolidone.

Severely ill chicks are best culled as, even if they recover, the check they receive will be sufficient to make them an uneconomic proposition. At the same time all efforts should be made to improve the management and general conditions of the remainder.

PREVENTION AND CONTROL

Prevention of yolk sac infection is very much a case of keeping hatching eggs as clean as possible and keeping the numbers of bacteria in the environment of the egg as low as possible. These objectives must be met from the time the egg is laid until after the chick is hatched.

1. Hatching eggs should be obtained from healthy stock, fed an adequate well balanced ration and maintained under good conditions of housing, hygiene and management.
2. Nest boxes should be kept in a clean condition and eggs collected as soon as possible after laying. Floor laid eggs should not be used for hatching.
3. Where eggs are stored on the farm the egg room should be kept clean and tidy. The temperature should be 55°-60°F (12.7°-15.5°C) and the relative humidity 75 per cent.
4. Eggs should not be stored for more than seven days before setting.
5. As soon as possible after laying, all eggs should be fumigated by the formalin, potassium permanganate method. This may be repeated at the hatchery prior to setting.
6. At the hatchery the strictest attention should be paid to maintaining a high standard of hygiene. All dust and debris must be regularly removed from hatchery rooms, incubators and hatchers and all equipment should be washed and disinfected as frequently as possible.
7. Incubators, hatchers and egg rooms should be fumigated as a routine when empty.
8. A thorough terminal disinfection between hatches should always be performed.
9. After hatching the chicks must be handled as little as possible. Sexing should be carried out quickly and efficiently.
10. The chicks should be transported as rapidly and efficiently as possible, avoiding long delays, draughts and other stresses, to the brooding site where the standards of housing, feeding and management should be as high as possible.

It must be borne in mind that stressing of chicks may convert a potential yolk sac infection into an actual one. Prevention of stress factors is therefore essential if yolk sac infection and other neo-natal conditions are to be avoided.

CHAPTER 7

Colisepticaemia

A MODERN DISEASE

A typical example of a disease, the incidence of which has increased dramatically with increasing intensivism in the poultry industry, is **colisepticaemia**. Almost unknown in the days when poultry were reared in small numbers under free range conditions, the disease increased in incidence to become one of the major obstacles to development of an intensive broiler industry. Although the disease is now as a rule adequately controlled by improved hygiene, better environmental control and reduction of the incidence of other precipitating respiratory disease, together with antibiotic treatment, it can still cause severe losses in individual cases, particularly where therapy is not commenced early in the course of the disease.

Chickens, particularly broilers, and turkeys are mainly affected, but outbreaks also occur in intensively reared ducks and occasionally in game-birds.

CAUSE AND PREDISPOSING FACTORS

Colisepticaemia is caused by various strains of the bacterial organism *Escherichia coli*. These organisms are present in large numbers in the environment of any poultry house and, indeed, live in the intestines of birds and other animals without causing any disease. Certain strains, however, have disease-causing potential and these have a tendency to localise in the birds' upper respiratory tract. An outbreak of disease is then liable to occur depending on the health and resistance of the birds and the presence of other

42

respiratory disease, e.g., Newcastle disease, infectious bronchitis or mycoplasmosis. The presence of these primary infections appears to "weaken" the birds' respiratory defence mechanisms and allow invasion of the blood stream by the pathogenic *E.coli*, i.e., colisepticaemia. It should be noted that live virus vaccination against Newcastle disease and infectious bronchitis can act as the precipitating factor for outbreaks of colisepticaemia, a fact which has somewhat reduced the attractiveness of this disease control method for some broiler growers.

Other factors which may predispose to outbreaks of the disease are lack of adequate ventilation, high concentrations of ammonia in the atmosphere and overcrowding. In addition, birds may be more susceptible to the infection where their vitality is reduced by such diseases as coccidiosis or nutritional deficiency. Broiler growers in particular should be aware that *E. coli* is an ever-present threat to their flocks and may take advantage of any fault in management or reduction in health status of the birds.

Transmission

The original source of infection is probably *E.coli* organisms which are present in large numbers in the environment. These cause a respiratory infection, and environmental contamination is then further increased by coughing and sneezing of large numbers of organisms into the atmosphere. By this means infection rapidly spreads throughout a poultry house. It was formerly believed that in some cases colisepticaemia followed invasion of a pathogenic strain of *E. coli* from the intestinal tract. This method of infection is now thought to occur rarely, if at all.

Signs

Colisepticaemia occurs most commonly in broilers of four to eight weeks of age, but outbreaks also occur in turkey poults and occasionally in pullet flocks. Sometimes the condition occurs in younger birds of about two weeks or less, and often in association with yolk sac infection.

Signs of colisepticaemia are mainly those of a respiratory infection although the degree of respiratory involvement will depend to some extent on the presence and effects of primary viral or other agents. Usually there is coughing and sneezing with respiratory distress but unless there is an accompanying mycoplasmal infection there is no facial swelling and little or no nasal discharge. Appetite is reduced, affected birds have a dejected appearance, growth and

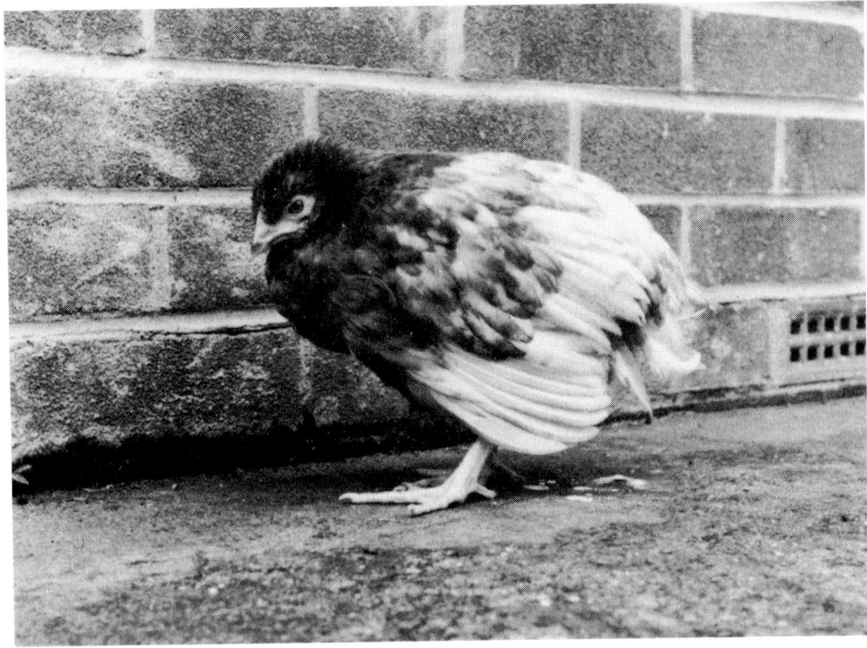

7.1   Colisepticaemia in seven week old pullet. A similar dejected appearance is seen in other conditions such as infectious synovitis.

food conversion are adversely affected and the incidence of condemnations and downgrading is increased when affected flocks are processed.

When younger flocks are affected a desire for increased heat may result in huddling under brooders sometimes with losses from smothering.

Mortality from colisepticaemia may vary from less than 2 per cent to over 20 per cent in severe cases. Signs of the disease are not specific and confirmation by post mortem examination is always necessary. It should be remembered that colisepticaemia is usually a secondary infection and the possibility of the presence of other respiratory infections or adverse environmental conditions should always be considered.

Post Mortem Findings

Of all diseases of poultry, colisepticaemia is perhaps the most easily diagnosed at post mortem. The carcase flesh often shows a reddish-purple discolouration, but the main changes are to be found on opening the carcase, on the heart and liver. The pericardium, or membrane surrounding the heart, which is normally a delicate transparent membrane, is thickened, white and opaque, and firmly adherent to the heart. The liver is covered by a thick white, opaque, deposit which is easily torn or broken, but which can with care be lifted cleanly off the liver in a continuous sheet. These changes are referred to as fibrinous pericarditis and perihepatitis. In addition the air sacs are often thickened and opaque and the film over the liver may extend to envelop the air sacs and cover the entire contents of the abdomen.

These changes are typical of colisepticaemia and are unlikely to be due to any other disease with the possible exception of a rare case of Salmonellosis. If confirmation is required *E.coli* can be easily isolated from the liver or heart in the laboratory.

Other changes associated with colisepticaemia are an enlarged dark liver, visible when the fibrin film is removed, enlarged spleen and a degree of tracheitis. It should be noted that not all these changes may be present in any one bird and that in some birds only slight pericarditis, for example, may be present. However, if a number of birds from an outbreak are examined, typical severe changes will probably be found in some of them and the diagnosis is not likely to be in doubt. Again, however, it must be stressed that colisepticaemia usually follows some other disease or adverse environmental influence and this should be sought and corrected as necessary.

Treatment

Colisepticaemia being a bacterial infection is treatable with antibiotics and other antibacterial substances. The most appropriate drug may be determined by sensitivity tests. Generally the **nitrofurans, furazolidone** and **furaltadone** are effective. The tetracyclines are also often used, as are ampicillin and spectinomycin. Neomycin, while theoretically effective, is not used because it is very poorly absorbed from the gut following oral administration.

If treatment is to be effective it must be started early in the course of an outbreak and adequate dose levels of drug used, whichever is chosen. Delay in treatment until the disease is well established and losses are high frequently results in poor response even at high drug dose levels.

PREVENTION AND CONTROL

Because of the ubiquitous nature of the causal organism, avoidance of infection is scarcely possible. Steps can be taken, however, to avoid actual disease. These include prevention of overcrowding, maintaining adequate ventilation and avoidance of high ammonia levels in the house. Attention to ventilation is particularly important as a means of lowering the numbers of organisms in the atmosphere. In many cases, especially in Winter, ventilation is reduced in order to maintain temperature. Provision of adequate insulation will go a long way to maintaining temperature without the necessity to reduce ventilation below required minimum levels.

Another important preventive measure, perhaps most important of all, is avoidance of infection by other respiratory pathogens. To this end vaccination against infectious bronchitis and Newcastle disease should be performed, although it is important to remember that the use of live virus vaccines result in a mild challenge of disease in the flock and this in itself may be sufficient to give rise to an outbreak of colisepticaemia. However, vaccination recommendations change, and it is now known that day-old vaccination of broilers against infectious bronchitis using a coarse spray technique gives adequate protection with no respiratory reaction. In the case of Newcastle Disease it is usual to administer only the milder **Hitchener B1** vaccine to broilers to avoid reaction from the more potent **La Sota**, except where there is a strong likelihood of occurrence of the disease in the flock, when both vaccines may be used. While vaccination against both diseases should be performed, the possibility of reaction, with secondary colisepticaemia should be borne in mind. The use of an antibiotic vitamin mix following vaccination may give some protection against adverse reaction.

The use of accepted hygiene standards and thorough cleaning, disinfection and fumigation of poultry houses following outbreaks may reduce the possibility of the infection occurring in subsequent crops.

CHAPTER 8

Avian Pasteurellosis

Avian pasteurellosis or **fowl cholera** is a bacterial disease of avian species which, in its most severe form, is one of the most acute and fatal of all poultry diseases. The disease occurs in fowls, turkeys, ducks and other birds, including game birds, in many countries of the world, but in its most acute form has not been seen in Britain for many years. When it did occur in the past, outbreaks could often be traced to imports of poultry from abroad. The term pasteurellosis also includes infection by *Pasteurella* (or *Yersinia*) *pseudotuberculosis*. This disease is considered briefly at the end of this chapter.

CAUSE

Pasteurellosis or fowl cholera is caused by a bacterial organism which has been given many names over the years but which is now usually referred to as *Pasteurella multicida*. Various strains occur, and the ability to cause disease depends on the strain involved and the species of bird infected. The organism is of historical interest in that Pasteur used it in his experiments on attenuation of bacteria for immunisation purposes.

OCCURRENCE AND COURSE OF THE DISEASE

Pasteurellosis occurs in various forms varying from extremely acute to mild and chronic, usually in adult birds or those approaching maturity. In turkey flocks it is seen almost invariably in birds of over eight weeks of age. In the most acute form the course is so rapid that birds are found dead without showing any signs of

47

illness. In less acute forms birds may be noticeably sick for several hours before death, while in the chronic type respiratory signs may be seen for a number of days or weeks before death or recovery occurs.

In one form of the disease infection is localised in the wattles, one or both of which are chronically swollen and inflamed.

It is generally agreed that certain environmental factors are important in determining the occurrence and severity of an outbreak. These include the nutritional status of the flock, the weather, the time of year and the state of hygiene of the premises. Outbreaks in turkeys, in particular, tend to occur on still, rather damp and misty days in Autumn, on premises on which hygiene standards are less than desirable and on which birds are overcrowded. The increased incidence in turkeys in Autumn may be partly due to the presence of large numbers of susceptible birds on farms at this time in preparation for the Christmas market.

TRANSMISSION

The source of infection in individual outbreaks of pasteurellosis can be difficult to determine, but it is well known that survivors of an outbreak may become chronic, symptomless carriers of the infection. These carriers shed the organism in their nasal and oral secretions and so contaminate their environment, including water and food, from which other birds then acquire the infection. Pasteurella organisms seldom survive passage through the digestive tract so that faecal contamination rarely occurs.

Wild birds may act as a source of the disease as may pigs, which are susceptible to infection by avian pasteurella organisms. Egg transmission is believed not to occur.

Following the introduction of the disease to a susceptible flock, further dissemination occurs by airborne transmission of material coughed from infected birds. The disease may also be spread between birds and between flocks by the use of contaminated crates, feed bags and other equipment or by human attendants.

Signs

The signs shown depend on the type of disease. In the per-acute form there are usually no ante-mortem signs of disease, birds being found dead in the cages or on the floor. In rather less acute forms birds appear mopey, with ruffled feathers, stand apart from the rest of the flock and refuse food and water. There may be diarrhoea and discharge from the nostrils, eyes and mouth. Death generally occurs in a number of hours, or up to a day or two after signs are first shown, although some birds may recover slowly. Chronic pasteurellosis may be a sequel to the acute disease, but is usually due to infection with a less virulent strain of the organism. The signs are mainly those of a respiratory infection, with coughing, ocular and nasal discharge and some difficulty in breathing. Sometimes there is lameness due to infection of joints, or twisting of the neck due to middle ear infection.

The wattle form of pasteurellosis is a type of chronic disease in which infection is localised in the wattles. It is often seen in cocks and is probably due to infection of wounds following fighting. One or both wattles may be affected and in the early stages are swollen, red, hot and painful — later they become pale and shrunken. Outbreaks of acute disease do not normally follow this form of infection.

Mortality in pasteurellosis may vary from almost nil in chronic disease to 90 per cent or more in the per-acute form in susceptible birds.

Post Mortem Findings

These also vary with the type of disease. In the per-acute form minute haemorrhages are seen scattered over the internal organs particularly the gizzard, heart, small intestine and abdominal fat. There may be some fluid in the pericardial sac and the carcase may have a fevered appearance, but the changes are not specific for pasteurellosis.

In the acute form these changes are accompanied by swelling of the liver with pin-point foci of necrosis throughout its substance and usually some evidence of pneumonia and pleurisy. The respiratory changes are particularly evident in turkeys, in which one or both lungs are almost completely solidified, the normal pink colour being changed to a patchy reddish-grey with yellow purulent foci in the substance of the lungs. In no other disease are such severe lung changes likely to be seen. In view of this severe pneumonia with progression to a stage of almost total solidification of the lungs, it is remarkable that birds so affected may show respiratory signs for only a very short time before death.

Severe pneumonia also occurs in pasteurellosis in ducks. In chronic pasteurellosis respiratory changes are also evident with lung congestion, extensive pleurisy and air sacculitis, the precise changes depending on the strain of organism involved and the degree of secondary infection. Birds lose weight and the comb and wattles are pale or bluish and shrunken. In localised forms of the disease there may be swelling or shrinking of the wattles, purulent fluid in and around the joints, swelling of the facial sinuses or purulent foci in various other locations.

Diagnosis

Although the signs, post mortem appearance and character of an outbreak may suggest pasteurellosis these are not specific for the disease. Per-acute pasteurellosis could, for example, be confused with acute erysipelas. Hence it is essential that the organism be isolated and identified in the laboratory to confirm the diagnosis.

Treatment

Per-acute cholera outbreaks are generally so explosive that attempts at treatment are ineffective although some birds may be saved by putting the flock on sulphaquinoxaline in the drinking water. In acute outbreaks this type of treatment is generally very effective, deaths stopping soon after commencement of treatment. If visibly sick birds are injected with antibiotic, preferably tetracycline, some of these may recover. It should be stated that where sulphaquinoxaline treatment is used, outbreaks may recur following withdrawal of treatment. Repeat treatment may be necessary, or in turkey flocks the drug may be given on a preventive basis, one day in every four or five, until the birds are ready for killing.

In chronic disease, treatment with injectable antibiotics may be tried but the effect may be disappointing. This is also the case in localised infections. Killing and disposal of affected birds is probably the best way of dealing with these cases.

PREVENTION AND CONTROL

The carrier bird as the main source of infection of pasteurellosis must be borne in mind when planning preventive measures. Obviously mixing of birds of different ages or from different sources should be avoided. The danger of infection being introduced by wild birds or acquired from pigs should also be considered. As in other infectious diseases, high standards of hygiene are important in preventing the disease. As mentioned earlier, outbreaks tend to occur on premises where hygiene standards are low. Prevention of contamination of feed and water sources is particularly important.

Vaccines are now available for prevention of the disease in turkeys either singly or as a combined pasteurella-erysipelas vaccine. The degree of protection given by vaccination varies depending on the strain of organism which may infect the flock. As in the case of erysipelas it is likely that a turkey producer whose unprotected flock has experienced an outbreak of pasteurellosis will not fail to vaccinate succeeding flocks even if the degree of protection afforded is not one hundred per cent.

Pseudotuberculosis.

This condition, caused by an organism known as *Pasteurella pseudotuberculosis*, or in more modern terms, *Yersinia pseudotuberculosis*, occurs on rare occasions in poultry. Turkey flocks are mainly affected. It is a common disease of canaries, other cage birds and wild birds, particularly of the finch family, and also of rodents. These probably constitute the main source of infection for poultry. Unlike *Pasteurella multicida* infection, organisms are passed in the droppings and infection occurs by ingestion of these infected droppings or by organisms gaining entry through skin wounds.

Signs of the disease are inconstant. Sudden death early in the course of the disease may occur, but, more commonly, birds become chronically affected, with diarrhoea and loss of weight being the main signs. Mortality is usually low, but occasional severe outbreaks in young turkey flocks have been recorded.

Post mortem findings are rather constant and consist of enlargement of the liver and spleen with multiple yellow-white necrotic foci or nodules throughout these organs. Sometimes the lungs and other organs are similarly affected. The lesions in the liver and spleen bear a strong resemblance to tuberculosis, hence the name pseudo (or false) tuberculosis. Bacteriological examination in the laboratory is often necessary to distinguish the two diseases.

Treatment of the disease is not usually undertaken, but where losses are persistent tetracycline antibiotics may give some success. Prevention depends largely on improved hygiene and keeping wild birds and rodents out of contact with poultry flocks.

CHAPTER 9

Staphylococcal Infections

BACTERIAL ORGANISMS

Staphylococci are common and widely distributed bacterial organisms which cause a variety of clinical conditions in many animal species, including man. In poultry they are responsible for a form of lameness, known as Staphylococcal arthritis (or "Bumblefoot" when the feet are affected) and other occasional and sporadic conditions including:

1. Skin and wound infections
2. Breast blister infections
3. Infection of the heart valves
4. A generalised infection or septicaemia.

They are also occasionally involved in yolk sac infection in baby chicks and are believed to play a part in gangrenous dermatitis.

Staphylococci are commonly found in the skin and upper respiratory tissues of chickens where normally they cause no ill effects, only becoming pathogenic and invading the tissues, or occasionally the blood stream, when the skin is injured or bruised, or when the bird is subjected to conditions of stress. The pathogenic species of Staphylococcus is *S.aureus*. Also commonly found in the environment and skin of chickens is *S.albus*; this organism, however, is generally considered non-pathogenic.

STAPHYLOCOCCAL ARTHRITIS.

This is one of the commoner causes of lameness in poultry, occurring in broilers, pullets, turkeys and broiler breeders, particularly during rearing. It is most often seen in birds on litter, but can also occur in cages, particularly where rough surfaces or wire projections are not attended to which may injure birds' feet.

Cause

The condition is caused by *Staphylococcus aureus* which invades the tissues or blood stream, following injury to the skin, especially of the feet. The infection then tends to localise in the joints, tendons and adjacent tissues. Any environmental factor which may result in skin injury; e.g., sharp projections, wood splinters in litter, or birds suffering injury when rushing to feeders where feed restriction is practised (in broiler breeders particularly) will result in an increased incidence of the condition. Since the organism is prevalent in the environment, bird to bird spread infection is not of importance.

Signs

The main sign of Staphylococcal arthritis is lameness of one or both legs and reluctance to move. Hot painful swellings appear on the legs, especially in the region of the hock joint, also commonly on the toes and on the foot-pad when the condition is called Bumblefoot. Affected birds appear dejected and loss of condition and eventual emaciation occur, probably due to a combination of pain from the condition itself and failure of birds to find food and water as they become more lame. Some birds may die in the early acute stage of the condition; others in the chronic stage, some from starvation as they fail to reach food. A number of birds may make a partial recovery, but are left with chronically affected joints and are unlikley to achieve acceptable levels of production.

Mortality is variable but does not usually exceed 10 per cent and is often much lower.

Post Mortem Findings

Swollen joints, foot pads and peritendonous tissues are apparent on post mortem examination. Incision into these lesions shows the presence of cream-coloured purulent fluid. In chronically affected birds this fluid becomes dried and thickened and joint cavities contain caseous debris. Fibrous tissue may be laid down around affected joints. In the early stages, the liver may be swollen and contain necrotic foci. In chronic cases there are no visible changes in internal organs.

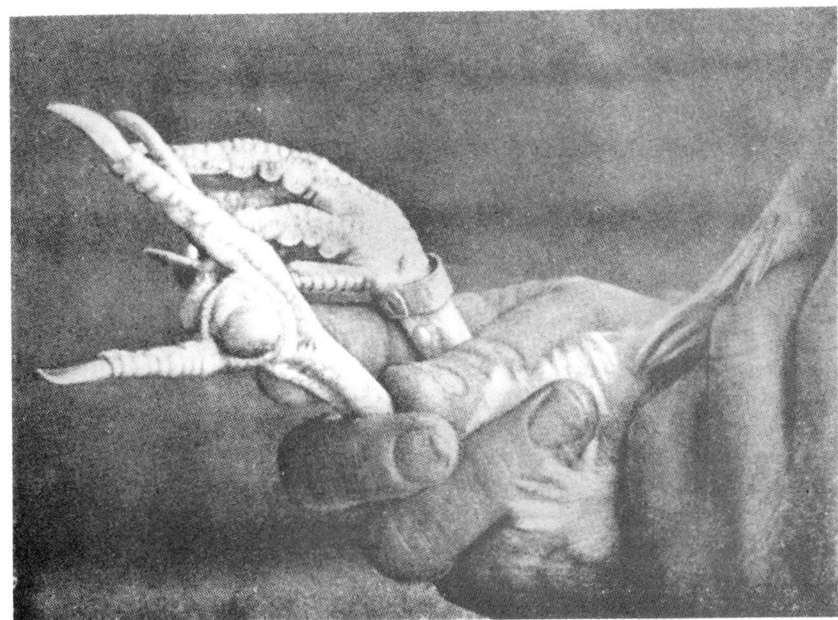

9.1   Bumble Foot: note the swelling on the inside of the foot. This is very painful and causes lameness.

Diagnosis

The disease should be suspected from the clinical signs and post-mortem changes but the condition cannot be differentiated from other conditions, particularly infectious synovitis, on gross post mortem. Confirmation of diagnosis depends on bacteriological examination of purulent fluid from lesions and recovery of *Staphylococcus aureus*.

TREATMENT

Treatment of Staphylococcal arthritis is by use of antibiotics including **Penicillin, Tetracyclines, Ampicillin** and **Streptomycin**. It is important that the most appropriate antibiotic is determined by sensitivity testing as many isolates are resistant to one or more antibiotics.

It should be said that antibiotic treatment sometimes gives disappointing results in the treatment of this disease probably due to inefficient contact of the antibiotic with the causative organisms. A prolonged course of antibiotic in the feed often gives best results. Severely affected birds are unlikely to recover and should be culled.

PREVENTION

High standards of hygiene may help to reduce numbers of Staphylococcal organisms in the environment. The most important factor in prevention, however, is the avoidance of any conditions which may cause injuries to the skin or feet. In the modern poultry industry, in which flocks number many thousands of birds, this objective may be impossible to achieve and occasional outbreaks of Staphylococcal arthritis are probably almost unavoidable. Vaccines against Staphylococci are not yet available.

CHAPTER 10

Clostridial Infections

MAIN CONDITIONS

The **clostridia** are a group of large (by microscopic standards) spore-forming bacterial organisms responsible for a number of conditions in a variety of animal species. In poultry they are responsible for three main conditions:
1. Botulism
2. Gangrenous dermatitis
3. Necrotic enteritis.

These are described in the sections which follow.

BOTULISM.

This condition is relatively rare in poultry and other animal species, but is not uncommon in waterfowl. It is well known as a rare, but extremely serious disease of man, usually acquired by eating spoiled tinned meat.

Cause

The disease is caused by a toxin produced in the course of multiplication of the bacterial organism *Clostridium botulinum*. This organism is common in nature but multiplication and toxin production occur only in rotting material, carcases, spoiled meat and vegetables, etc.. It is important to emphasise that the organism itself is not a cause of disease and its isolation from intestinal content, for example, is of no significance in disease diagnosis. The toxin it produces however is one of the most powerful poisons known. Several types of botulinus toxin are produced, the type which usually affects chickens being different from that which affects humans. It is unlikely therefore that an outbreak of food poisoning in humans would result from the consumption of contaminated chicken meat, particularly as the toxin is heat labile and would be destroyed by cooking.

Source of Outbreaks.

Botulism in broiler chickens is believed to be the result of birds ingesting toxin formed by growth of the organism in decaying carases which have not been removed from the house. The tendency of birds to peck at such material is well known. In the more frequent cases of poisoning in waterfowl the source of toxin is generally the bodies of slugs, snails, frogs or other aquatic creatures which have died and lie in or around ponds. Mortality of such pond-life apparently increases during a period of hot weather when water levels in ponds tends to fall and the carcases are a suitable medium for growth of *Clostridium botulinum*. Maggots feeding on carcases may contain sufficient toxin to poison birds if they in turn are eaten. Toxin can also be found in rotting vegetable material and in rotting carcases of birds which have been shot or have died due to other causes.

Signs

The botulinus toxin affects principally the nervous system and signs are those of weakness and inco-ordination progressing to paralysis of neck, wing and legs followed by coma and death. The condition has been called "limberneck" from the usual initial paralysis of the neck. In some cases an additional sign is looseness of the feathers which may fall out if birds are handled or disturbed.

Birds may begin to show signs within a few hours of ingestion of toxin. If significant quantities of toxin are consumed by many birds mortality may be considerable. Death is usually rapid and the whole outbreak may be over in a number of days.

Diagnosis

There are no post mortem findings in birds dead of botulism. Diagnosis depends on demonstration of a possible source of toxin, close observation of signs and extraction of toxin from the digestive tracts of birds showing signs, or those which have died. Injection of toxin into mice in the laboratory, resulting in paralysis or death of those unprotected, and survival of those protected by antitoxin, confirms the diagnosis

Prevention

In the case of broilers daily removal of carcases of birds which have died will eliminate the commonest medium for growth of the organism and elaboration of the toxin. Removal of all sources of toxin from ponds is impractical, but individual waterfowl showing signs may be saved by injection of antitoxin. Removal of birds from ponds at danger times may be possible in some circumstances.

GANGRENOUS DERMATITIS

This relatively new disease occurs mainly in broilers and is characterised by discoloration and oedema of the skin and sub-cutaneous tissues in various areas of the body, including the wings. As a result it has also been called "Wing-rot".

The condition or a similar disease was described as long ago as 1939 under the name Vesicular Dermatitis. A number of reports followed, but only in the last ten years has it become a condition of economic significance. Although seen most commonly in broilers, of five to seven weeks of age, it also occurs in pullet flocks and turkey poults.

Cause and Source of Outbreaks

Gangrenous dermatitis is a bacterial infection of subcutaneous tissues and underlying muscles caused by the bacterial organism *Clostridium septicum. Staphylococcus aureus* is also believed to be involved, but the disease has not been reproduced with this organism alone and its role in the disease is still uncertain.

It should be understood that both clostridia and staphylococci occur widely in nature and in the environment of the chicken. Clostridia can frequently be isolated from intestinal content and staphylococci from skin, and isolation is not in itself indicative of disease. It appears that some form of tissue injury *must* occur for these organisms to be transformed from harmless commensals to the pathogenic state. This tissue injury may be simple physical damage due to high stocking densities or nutritional deficiency, particularly of Vitamin E or Selenium. Tissue damage resulting from these or other causes favours growth of opportunist organisms which may be present.

There appears to be a causal relationship between infectious bursal disease and other conditions, including inclusion body hepatitis and gangrenous dermatitis, in that infectious bursal disease by depressing immune mechanisms and lowering antibody production, impairs the bird's ability to withstand such conditions. The importance of these disease inter-relationships under field conditions is still the subject of investigation.

Signs

There are no particular signs associated with gangrenous dermatitis in the live bird. If seen before death, affected birds are dull, with reduced appetite and possibly increased thirst. Generally, however, the condition comes to light when birds are found dead, showing the characteristic lesions.

Post Mortem Findings

The skin of the thighs, wings, back, breast and sometimes the shanks and feet shows blue-black discoloration suggestive of severe bruising. The skin on affected areas can be easily removed to show blood-tinged fluid and bubbles of gas in the subcutaneous tissues. The muscular tissues are dark red or almost black in colour and haemorrhagic. The skin of the shanks and feet, where these are affected, peels off easily and the foot pad may be ruptured. In some birds the liver is swollen and discoloured with necrotic foci in its substance and the bone marrow may be pale. It may be noticed that rapid degeneration or "rotting" of the carcase takes place following death.

The above description refers to **severe cases** of gangrenous dermatitis. In many birds lesions may be much less severe and in these cases care must be taken to differentiate between true cases of gangrenous dermatitis and skin damage due to bruising, treading by other birds while carcases have lain on the floor, or other similar causes of skin discoloration.

Mortality in gangrenous dermatitis outbreaks is variable, but in severe outbreaks may be 30 per cent of the flock.

Diagnosis

A diagnosis in most cases can be made from the distinctive lesions. In doubtful cases birds should be submitted to a laboratory for bacteriological examination. Isolation of the causal organisms from lesions tends to support the diagnosis, although the prevalence of these organisms in the chicken's environment must be borne in mind.

Treatment

Antibiotics including **tetracyclines** and **penicillin** may be used to treat gangrenous dermatitis. **Sulphaquinoxaline** however has been found to be highly effective and is now used in preference to antibiotics. Birds in advanced stages of the disease are unlikely to recover whatever treatment is used.

PREVENTION

Because gangrenous dermatitis often occurs on farms where hygiene levels are less than desirable an improved level of hygiene may help to prevent further outbreaks. Clostridia are more susceptible to the action of iodine based disinfectants than phenolic or cresylic compounds and it is important that these should be used for disinfection following outbreaks.

An association between infectious bursal disease and gangrenous dermatitis has already been mentioned. Infectious bursal disease, by its action on the cloacal bursa, suppresses immune mechanisms including circulating antibody production. It has been found that vaccination against infectious bursal disease indirectly protects against gangrenous dermatitis by preventing immuno-suppression so that the bird is able to mount a full antibody response to the disease. On farms with a history of gangrenous dermatitis this has proved to be a useful preventive measure.

NECROTIC ENTERITIS

Necrotic enteritis is a bacterial infection of the intestine mainly of broilers of between two and six weeks of age. It is not a particularly common condition, but is of some importance because of the high mortality it can cause and due to the possibility of its being confused with coccidiosis.

Cause

Necrotic enteritis is caused primarily by infection of the intestine with the bacterial organism *Clostridium welchii* type A or type C. It has not, however, been possible consistently to reproduce the disease by administration of cultures of this organism and other predisposing factors are believed to operate. Chief of these is probably coccidiosis infection particularly with *Eimeria maxima* or *E. brunetti*. These types of coccidiosis appear to alter conditions within the bowel so that growth of, and toxin production by Clostridia are increased. Dietary factors may also play a part; the condition apparently tends to occur when normal bowel motility is slowed down as may result from lack of fibre in the diet.

Signs

Birds suffering from necrotic enteritis are dull, depressed, off their food and may have dark coloured diarrhoea. Signs, however, are not characteristic and may be confused with other conditions, particularly coccidiosis.

Mortality is variable but may be 30 per cent of a flock or more in untreated outbreaks. Where appropriate treatment is instituted early, losses will be much less.

Post Mortem Findings

In birds dead of necrotic enteritis the main changes are found in the intestine. The lower small intestine is mainly affected, but in some cases the entire length of bowel from duodenum to large intestine may be involved. The bowel is distended and the contents are a dirty brown-coloured liquid or semi-solid, foul-smelling material. Removal of this material will show the bowel wall to be thickened, brown-stained, devitalised or necrotic in appearance. In many areas there is irregular, patchy sloughing of the mucous membrane, leaving a somewhat ragged mucosal surface.

In some affected birds there are necrotic foci in the liver and in more chronic cases there may be varying degrees of loss of condition.

DIAGNOSIS & TREATMENT

The post mortem changes are rather characteristic and diagnosis can generally be made accurately from these. If confirmation is required, laboratory bacteriological examination of the intestine to demonstrate causative Clostridial bacteria will be necessary. These may be found in the large intestine, but not in the small intestine, in normal birds. These organisms are highly susceptible to penicillin and treatment with soluble penicillin in the drinking water usually effects rapid cure.

In some cases microscopic examination of bowel scrapings will show variable numbers of coccidial oocysts and there may be some doubt as to which is the more severe condition requiring more urgent treatment. As a rule, if typical necrotic enteritis is present, a short (two day) course of penicillin treatment followed by treatment for coccidiosis will give satisfactory control of both conditions.

PREVENTION

Because Clostridia are prevalent in the environment little can be done to prevent the condition other than application of rigorous hygiene standards. Since coccidiosis and necrotic enteritis are often associated, prevention of the former condition may help also to prevent the latter.

CHAPTER 11

Erysipelas

NATURE OF DISEASE

Although **erysipelas** is principally a disease of pigs it also occurs in man and many other animal species. In birds it has been seen in chickens, turkeys, ducks, geese, pigeons, game and wild birds. In Britain, however, it is only in turkeys that it assumes any economic importance.

Erysipelas is a bacterial infection, caused by an organism known as *Erysipelothrix rhusiopathiae,* which is fairly widely distributed in nature and can live in soil and decaying matter for long periods. It is commonly found in the throat and gut of healthy pigs and, to a less extent, in these regions in other animals. Despite the fact that *Erysipelothrix rhusiopathiae* can live for long periods outside the animal body it is fairly readily killed by disinfectants employed in the strengths recommended for general use, as well as by heat. The exact portal of entry of the organism into the turkey's body is still uncertain, but it is generally believed that cuts and abrasions in the skin are the main route of infection. Infection by mouth is probably also important.

Birds of between three and seven months most often contract erysipelas but both younger and older stock can be affected. Male birds are apparently more susceptible than females, but this may be a consequence of the male habit of fighting which results in injuries to the skin allowing entry of the organism. Other "stress factors" also apparently increase the susceptibility of turkeys to erysipelas. These may include overcrowding, damp or inclement weather, sudden changes of temperature and poor hygienic conditions.

63

SYMPTOMS

At the beginning of an outbreak one or two birds are usually found dead without having previously shown any apparent signs of ill-health. Later some may be seen looking dejected, standing about with lowered head, drooping wings and ruffled feathers. Affected turkeys usually have little or no appetite and a greenish-yellow diarrhoea is sometimes present. The snood is often swollen and purplish blotches may be noted on the skin, particularly in the head and breast regions. Generally, birds either die or have recovered within ten days from the onset of symptoms. A few, however, may linger, becoming progressively thinner and eventually dying. The death rate varies greatly, from as low as one or two birds to as high as 75 per cent of the flock. In the most acute cases a characteristic of the disease is very high mortality with no premonitory signs.

Post Mortem Findings

There are no characteristic changes in the internal organs of turkeys that have died from erysipelas. However pin-point or slightly larger haemorrhages on the surface of the heart, gizzard, abdominal and pleural membranes and other organs as well as in the carcase musculature, are usually easily visible in some birds that have died in the course of an outbreak. Such haemorrhages in turkeys following sudden death should give rise to suspicion of erysipelas. In addition the liver, spleen and kidneys may be somewhat enlarged and there may be a mucoid enteritis. The snood is sometimes reddish-purple in colour and swollen or turgid.

These changes are not, however, diagnostic of erysipelas and in order to establish a diagnosis fresh carcases should be submitted to a laboratory where the causative organism can be cultured from internal organs. Isolation of the organism serves to distinguish the disease from other conditions, especially Pasteurellosis or fowl cholera, which can also cause sudden death in turkeys.

PREVENTION AND CONTROL

Since erysipelas is a common disease of pigs it must be borne in mind that where pigs and turkeys are reared on the same premises the possibility of outbreaks of erysipelas occurring in the turkeys is somewhat increased. Under these circumstances it is essential to vaccinate the birds against the disease using one of the several efficient vaccines which are now on the market. Indeed, it is suggested that all turkey flocks should be vaccinated against erysipelas. Where the disease occurs in an unprotected flock, unless treatment can be started rapidly, losses are likely to be such as to cause a good deal of regret in the mind of the flock owner that he left the birds unvaccinated, and it is unlikely that he will fail to take this precaution on future occasions.

Vaccination is administered by injection at 8-10 weeks of age; i.e., before the age at which the disease is usually contracted. Two injections are given at an interval of two weeks.

When an outbreak occurs treatment is by means of **antibiotics**, of which penicillin is most effective. Because of the possible acuteness of the disease and high death rate treatment must be instituted early in the course of an outbreak. A rapid acting penicillin injection should be given to all birds in the flock and treatment continued for several days by soluble penicillin in the drinking water. Since the organism is highly sensitive to penicillin this regimen usually gives good results, but a close watch must be kept on the flock, as a second outbreak can occur at a later date, particularly if it is not possible to move the birds to fresh ground after an outbreak. Where the flock has to be maintained on the same contaminated ground, vaccination at the same time as the original penicillin injection would be advisable. It must be emphasised that the organism can live in soil for long periods of time and where a flock is placed on ground previously occupied by birds in which an outbreak occurred, even if an interval of several months is allowed to elapse, vaccination of that flock is a wise precaution.

Finally it must be remembered that erysipelas produces painful infections in man, the organism usually gaining entry through cuts or scratches on the fingers. Care should be taken to protect the hands when handling birds in which erysipelas has occurred or is suspect.

Note: Erysipelas of turkeys and pigs should not be confused with **human erysipelas** which is caused by a member of the Streptococcus genus of bacteria. This is a severe generalised infection of man. The localised infection on the hands of humans caused by the turkey erysipelas organism is correctly referred to as **erysipeloid**.

CHAPTER 12

Other Bacterial Infections

AVIAN ARIZONA INFECTION

The **Arizona** group of bacteria are closely related to the Salmonella or paratyphoid organisms described in a previous chapter. The disease they cause is also in many ways identical to that caused by the Salmonellae. It is an important condition in the U.S.A. and many other countries, but has been recorded only once in Britain in a batch of turkeys imported from America.

Arizonosis occurs mainly in turkeys, in which it causes clinical signs of general malaise, listlessness and huddling, inappetance and diarrhoea. In addition, nervous signs of twisted necks, leg paralysis and convulsions are frequently present and some poults become blind in one or both eyes. As in salmonellosis transmission occurs either vertically or by lateral spread. Adult birds act as sources of infection for chicks, but seldom show any clinical evidence of disease.

Post Mortem Findings

Post mortem findings again are similar to those of salmonellosis and include enlarged livers which may be yellowish or mottled, infected yolk sacs, generalised peritonitis, pericarditis and caseous caecal cores. In blind birds the eye surface is covered by a white caseous deposit.

Diagnosis of Arizona infection depends on recovery of the causative organism in the laboratory. The signs and post mortem changes do not distinguish it from salmonellosis. Infected flocks may be treated by furazolidone in the feed or furaltadone in the drinking water as for salmonellosis. Known infected flocks should not however be retained for breeding purposes because of the difficulty in eliminating carrier birds.

Control

Control methods are identical to those for salmonellosis and depend mainly on hygiene methods on the breeding farm and in the hatchery, and prevention of contamination of the shell of the hatching egg. Blood tests for detecting adult carriers have been used but are not entirely satisfactory.

INFECTIOUS CORYZA

This is a bacterial infection of the respiratory system caused by the organism *Haemophilus gallinarum*. It is of significance only in chickens, although cases rarely occur in pheasants. All ages may be affected, but the disease is more common and severe in adult birds. At present it is almost non-existent in Britain, but is important in many other countries including certain states of the U.S.A..

Infectious coryza is an infection of the respiratory tract, particularly of the upper tract and the main signs are swelling of the face, mucous discharge from the eyes and nostrils, conjunctivitis, sneezing and in some cases swelling of the wattles. When the lower respiratory tract is involved there is gurgling and difficulty in breathing. Appetite is lost and growth rate or egg production are adversely affected.

The severity of signs and mortality, which may vary from almost nil up to 20 per cent or more, apparently depend on the virulence of the infecting organism and the presence of other intercurrent infections. The uncomplicated disease has a short course whereas if other infections such as *Mycoplasma gallisepticum* or fowl pox complicate the picture, chronic disease lasting for a number of weeks may result. Recovered birds remain carriers and constitute the main source of infection for other birds or flocks.

Post Mortem Findings

Post mortem findings include a generalised inflammatory reaction of the upper respiratory tract. In uncomplicated disease there is usually little evidence of caseation in the trachea or sinuses, but subcutaneous oedema (accumulation of fluid under the skin) will be evident on incising the skin of the face or wattles. Diagnosis depends on laboratory isolation of the organism since the disease may be confused with other respiratory infections. It should be remembered that other infections often occur concurrently with coryza and this should be taken into account when making a diagnosis.

Treatment

Various antibiotics and sulphonamides have been used for treatment of the condition and some improvement on a flock basis can be expected. However, a recurrence of disease often occurs after cessation of treatment and the carrier state is not eliminated. Some of the more successful antibiotics used are **erythromycin**, **spectinomycin** and **oxytetracycline**.

Prevention

Prevention of the disease depends on rearing of chicks away from carrier bird sources of infection and use of hygiene precautions as in other infectious diseases. Vaccination may be used in countries where the disease is endemic, but no vaccine is available or necessary in Britain. Vaccines are generally administered by injection, two injections being given between ten and twenty weeks of age, with a three week interval. This regime gives satisfactory protection against drops in egg production and mortality from the disease.

VIBRIONIC HEPATITIS.

This is a disease of some importance in certain states of the U.S.A., in Germany, Italy and several other countries, but it is rare in Britain. It is caused by a bacterial organism of the *Vibrio* genus.

The disease occurs almost exclusively in chickens, particularly in pullets coming into lay. It is spread mainly by elimination of organisms in faeces, infection of other birds readily occurring by ingestion. The infection becomes established in the intestines and spreads to involve the liver. The disease runs a prolonged, chronic course, slowly spreading through a flock over a period of weeks or months. Signs include loss of condition, pale comb and wattles, listlessness and diarrhoea. In laying birds there may be a severe drop in egg production.

Detection

Post mortem changes mainly involve the liver which in recent cases is enlarged, pale in colour with necrotic foci or haemorrhages visible on its surface. Sometimes large areas of necrosis are present and in long-standing cases almost the entire liver may be pale, shrunken and firm with little normal tissue remaining. Other changes include degeneration of the ovaries, enlargement of the spleen and heart, necrotic areas in the heart and varying degrees of enteritis. Mortality rates vary from almost nil to twenty per cent or more.

Signs and post mortem findings may be sufficient to give rise to suspicion of the disease, but confirmation requires isolation of the organism in the laboratory. This is most easily achieved from liver, bile or caeca.

Control

Antibiotic treatment gives some control of the disease, but in many cases is not totally effective and recurrence is not uncommon following withdrawal of treatment. **Furazolidone** appears to be the most effective anti-bacterial for treatment of vibrionic hepatitis.

Normal hygiene measures will help to prevent outbreaks of vibrionic hepatitis. Because it is often noted that other diseases or stress factors precede outbreaks of vibrionic hepatitis, maintaining the general health of susceptible flocks may help to avoid outbreaks of this disease.

CHAPTER 13

Avian Mycoplasmosis

NATURE OF DISEASES

Mycoplasma organisms are common infectious agents of poultry and other animals. Three species are important in poultry, namely *Mycoplasma gallisepticum*, *M. synoviae* in both chickens and turkeys and *M.meleagridis* in turkeys only.

The mycoplasma group of organisms may be regarded as being in many ways intermediate between viruses and bacteria. They were formerly known as P.P.L.O. or "pleuro-pneumonia-like-organisms". The disease syndrome produced by *M.gallisepticum* in chickens was known as chronic respiratory disease or C.R.D. although it was recognised that other organisms were also involved in the syndrome. As continuing work led to a better understanding of the respiratory disease complex the term C.R.D. became less meaningful and it is now seldom used. The disease conditions due to mycoplasmal infections should be referred to as *Mycoplasma gallisepticum* infection and *Mycoplasma meleagridis* infection. It is still acceptable to refer to *Mycoplasma synoviae* infection as infectious synovitis, although it should be noted that this organism can also cause respiratory disease similar to that caused by *M.gallisepticum*.

There is little doubt that avian mycoplasmas exist wherever poultry are kept and they have been a cause of considerable economic loss, particularly since the development of intensivism in the industry. The importance of these infections lies not only in their own disease producing ability, but also in the fact that their presence renders the respiratory system more susceptible to infection and damage by other disease-causing agents.

MYCOPLASMA GALLISEPTICUM INFECTION

As mentioned, this organism causes respiratory disease in chickens and turkey poults. It may also be responsible for slight dips in egg production graphs of laying flocks and occasionally it may be implicated in leg problems in chickens.

It should be stressed again, that when the organism is involved in severe respiratory disease this is usually the result of infection by other agents in addition to mycoplasmal infection. By itself *M. gallisepticum* generally gives rise to only mild disease signs, but frequently the infection is complicated by respiratory viruses or by *E.coli* infection when severe disease may result.

Spread of Infection

M.gallisepticum is transmitted through the egg from parents to offspring and also from bird to bird within a flock. Bird to bird transmission may be quite rapid within a flock but tends to be slow, or may not occur, between flocks or houses on a site. There is no doubt that egg transmission is the most important means of dissemination of the disease.

Signs

Mycoplasmosis is a condition mainly of the respiratory system and signs include coughing and "snicking", nasal discharge, watery eyes and conjunctivitis. In turkeys especially, but occasionally also in chickens, infection of the sinuses below the eyes can result in characteristic swellings on the side of the face which may result in closing of the eyes. One or both sinuses may be affected.

Depending on the severity of infection these signs may be quite marked or barely detectable. When other conditions complicate the picture, severe disease with high mortality may result. In uncomplicated disease mortality is usually low.

The signs just described are usually seen only in young or growing chicks or poults. In adults signs are usually mild and consist of slight eye or nasal discharge and occasional coughing and head shaking together with some loss of egg production. In many cases clinical signs may be so slight as to be undetectable the only evidence of infection being antibody production demonstrable by blood testing.

It is believed that *M. gallisepticum* is involved in some cases of infective leg problems and lameness in chickens.

Post Mortem Findings

In uncomplicated disease pathological changes are usually slight and confined to the respiratory tract. The most characteristic finding is flecks of white, caseous material adhering to the air sacs which may also be cloudy or frothy. There may also be some mucus in the nasal cavities and sinuses. In turkeys particularly, this mucus becomes caseous and solid giving rise to the facial swellings already mentioned. Incision into these swellings shows the solidified material filling the sinuses.

Diagnosis

The presence of typical clinical signs together with caseous material in the air sacs should give rise to suspicion of the disease. This is further supported by blood testing. Final confirmation of diagnosis requires isolation of *M.gallisepticum* in the laboratory but this is a difficult and time consuming exercise. The organism may take four weeks to grow and a negative result cannot be assumed earlier than this. Obviously a diagnosis will be required in most cases as soon as possible and a presumptive diagnosis may have to be made on signs, post mortem findings and blood testing. A plate test may be used but this, although rapid and convenient to perform, may not be sufficiently accurate for a number of reasons and the haemagglutination inhibition test, as for Newcastle Disease, should be used as a confirmatory test.

It should be noted that in some cases antibodies to *M.gallisepticum* may be detected on blood testing with no clinical signs in the birds. It cannot therefore, be assumed that respiratory signs in a flock are due to *M.gallisepticum* simply because antibodies are present in the blood. Further, secondary complicating disease, e.g. colisepticaemia may mask the presence of the less dramatic mycoplasmosis. It will be appreciated therefore that the precise diagnosis of mycoplasmosis and elucidation of its role in a respiratory disease outbreak may be matters of some difficulty.

Treatment

A number of antibiotics are available for treatment of outbreaks of Mycoplasma gallisepticum infection. These include **Erythromycin, Spiramycin, Tylosin** and **Spectinomycin** and may be given in the drinking water or by injection. While a good response to these antibiotics generally occurs it is not possible to ensure that infection is eliminated from all birds in the flock, so that subsequent outbreaks may occur. Also, if any other complicating disease is present, this may require additional treatment.

Control

Since *Mycoplasma gallisepticum* is egg transmitted, and lateral transmission from external sources occurs to only a limited extent, it should be possible to control and indeed totally eradicate the disease by prevention of egg transmission. Much effort has been put into this aspect of control by the breeding organisations and many now claim their stock to be Mycoplasma free.

Various methods have been used to eradicate the infection from breeding stock. These include antibiotic treatment of birds and of hatching eggs, and heat treatment of eggs. Antibiotic treatment of breeding birds will lower the level of infection of these birds and hence the number of infected eggs. Treatment of eggs then further reduces the numbers of infected eggs which hatch, and, consequently, the number of infected chicks or poults.

The usual method of introducing antibiotic into eggs is by immersing heated eggs in a cooled solution containing the antibiotic. Another method utilises pressure reducing apparatus, containing antibiotic solution into which eggs are placed, following which the pressure is allowed to return to normal. Both methods result in antibiotic being drawn through the shell into the egg where it comes in contact with Mycoplasmal organisms which may be present in the egg.

Heat treatment of eggs consists of heating eggs slowly to about 45°C (138°F) and, again, slowly lowering the temperature to normal. All these methods result in some loss from embryo mortality.

Eventually, if these bird and egg treatments are rigorously pursued freedom from infection will be established. Blood testing of breeder birds is performed to monitor freedom. If any birds are found positive for antibodies to the organism they are eliminated or the entire flock may be culled.

Generally, control methods for Mycoplasma applied to breeding flocks have given good results, yet infection in commercial flocks is not uncommon. This may be either clinical infection or detection of antibodies in the blood in the course of monitoring programmes. The origin of these infections can be difficult to explain, but when infection gains entry to a site it may be difficult to eradicate without total depopulation. There is no doubt that the reduction of infection by *Mycoplasma gallisepticum* of the poultry population has significantly improved the health of the national flock.

INFECTIOUS SYNOVITIS

Infectious synovitis is a disease of chickens and turkeys which was first recognised in America in 1954, affecting birds of four to twelve weeks of age in the broiler areas of the East, South and West. It has since been reported from many other countries and appears to be worldwide in distribution.

The disease, when it first appeared was seen only in broilers but now also occurs in pullet flocks and turkeys. It was a considerable problem to the broiler industry for a number of years, but its incidence has now been reduced by management and disease control measures.

Cause

The cause of the disease is a micro-organism belonging to the Mycoplasma group. The particular organism which causes infectious synovitis is called *Mycoplasma synoviae* and its main effect is in the joints and tendons causing a form of lameness, although it can also cause a mild respiratory condition.

Course and Spread of the Disease

Infectious synovitis occurs in broilers, pullets and turkeys, generally between four and sixteen weeks of age although older and younger birds can be affected. The disease may be divided into two stages, an acute stage in which birds are severely lame and depressed and a subsequent chronic stage during which a proportion of affected birds make a slow recovery. These recovered birds, however, remain carriers of infection and, in the case of breeding flocks, are capable of passing the organism to their offspring via the hatching egg. This appears to be the most important means of spread of the disease, but when infection is introduced in this way, spread from bird to bird by contact can occur quite readily, albeit rather slowly. Given time almost all birds in the flock may become infected although not all show signs of the disease. Such lateral spread appears to occur by way of the respiratory tract.

It has been found that separation of an infected flock from a clean flock by a wire partition may be enough to prevent spread of the disease between flocks, emphasising that direct contact is generally necessary for spread to occur. It would be unwise to assume that such a barrier would be effective in every case and, in fact, on some farms the disease, once it has been introduced, tends to become endemic, occurring in each flock until a complete "disease break" can be arranged.

It sometimes happens that infectious synovitis occurs in a flock of pullets of perhaps twelve to twenty weeks of age where no infection in the parent flock is suspected or can be detected. It can be difficult to determine the origin of such infection. The organism is known not to survive long outside the bird's body so that indirect transmission from an external source is unlikely. It may be that only a small number of chicks are infected via the egg from a few chronically infected and symptomless parents and that these chicks then pass the disease to their flock-mates. In order to detect the few infected parents, blood testing of all, or almost all, the parents would be necessary. While it is claimed that some breeding stock is free from *Mycoplasma synoviae* infection a good deal of infectious synovitis still occurs in commercial pullet and broiler flocks, and further work is required to establish the origin of these infections and to clarify certain aspects of spread of the disease which are not yet clearly understood.

Signs

Infectious synovitis is an infection of the joints, tendons and surrounding tissues, and signs are related to infection of these regions. Birds are unwilling to move and stand around with ruffled feathers and pale combs. They become lame and before long some go off their legs and sit on their hocks. Condition is rapidly lost, the birds becoming emaciated and dehydrated as they fail to reach food and water. Swellings around the hock joints or on the foot pads may be visible. Sometimes these swellings extend along the shank.

Recovery from infectious synovitis may occur, particularly if birds are able to reach food and water easily. Mortality from the disease is generally low. The condition may, however, progress to the chronic stage when the swellings disappear and birds recover use of their legs, but infection may not be eliminated so that some individuals become chronic carriers of the infection.

Post Mortem Findings and Diagnosis

Swellings in the regions of various joints are found in most infected birds in the acute stage. The hock joint and foot pad are most commonly affected, but wing joints are also often involved. Incision into the swellings shows an opaque, viscous, grey or cream coloured fluid in the joints and surrounding tissues. In the later stages this fluid tends to solidify and swellings become less obvious, and in the chronic stage affected tissues often acquire a yellowish or orange colour. In many cases breast blisters are present due to contact with the ground while the birds are off their legs, or due to the disease itself affecting this region.

There are few visible changes in the internal organs, but in some birds in the acute stage the liver, spleen and kidneys may be enlarged.

The mortality rate in infectious synovitis is not usually high and the main economic importance of this disease is the loss of condition and culling of affected broilers and pullets and the downgrading of broiler carcases due to the lesions just described.

The signs and post mortem changes are not specific for infectious synovitis and do not distinguish the disease from other conditions causing lameness. In particular they can be confused with Staphylococcal infections of the joints, and in order to establish a diagnosis affected birds should be sent to a laboratory where bacteriological examinations and blood testing can be performed. It should be mentioned that Mycoplasmas are particularly slow growing organisms on laboratory media and confirmation of their presence by cultural methods is difficult and time consuming. However, a positive blood test for antibodies to *Mycoplasma synoviae* together with failure to culture a *Staphylococcus* or other infection from joint fluid is strong evidence for the presence of infectious synovitis.

Treatment, Prevention and Control.

Mycoplasma synoviae is susceptible to antibiotics and treatment with chlortetracycline gives good results in preventing further cases in an infected flock. Prolonged treatment may be necessary to keep the disease under control. If treatment is stopped too early further cases may occur. Birds which are severely affected are unlikely to recover and should be culled.

Treatment of infected adult breeding flocks with antibiotic gives uncertain results and it is probably safer to stop hatching eggs from such flocks. However, much progress has been made in controlling the infection by means of blood testing of grandparent and parent flocks and eliminating birds in which antibodies to the organism are detected so preventing egg transmission of the disease. Different workers have recommended various testing schedules and numbers of birds to be tested within flocks and certain problems arise in interpretation of results. Further work is required to standardise these procedures and to iron out associated difficulties.

Other methods of controlling egg transmission of the disease have included heating of fertile eggs before incubation and treatment of fertile eggs with antibiotics both by egg-dipping and by injection of antibiotic into the eggs. Again both these procedures give rise to certain difficulties. Doubtless, however, continued work along these lines will eventually result in a poultry population free from this troublesome disease.

MYCOPLASMA MELEAGRIDIS INFECTION

Mycoplasma meleagridis infection is the third significant mycoplasmal infection of poultry but unlike *M.gallisepticum* and *M.synoviae* this species affects only turkeys. It was first described as a pathogen of turkeys in 1958 and with the declining incidence and importance of *M.gallisepticum* in recent years, *M.meleagridis* has emerged as an important and widely distributed cause of respiratory disease in turkeys. Efforts are now being made by a number of turkey breeding organisations to eliminate this organism from their stock by preventing egg transmission as has been achieved in the case of the other mycoplasmas.

Spread of Infection

The main means of transmission as in other mycoplasma infections is via the egg. *M.meleagridis* infection is in fact a true venereal disease, infection of the female occurring by means of insemination with contaminated semen. Infection of the reproductive tract is necessary for egg transmission to occur; birds in which infection is confined to the respiratory tract seldom transmit the organism to their offspring, although there is some evidence that infection may later move from the respiratory tissues to the reproductive system. The rate of egg transmission varies from bird to bird and may be from 10 to 50 per cent of eggs laid.

In a flock of poults in which a proportion of the birds have been infected via the egg, further spread can occur laterally on the hatcher trays or during brooding although the importance of such lateral spread under practical conditions has not been fully evaluated. Also the significance of lateral transmission between adult birds in contributing to genital infection is uncertain, but is believed to be relatively unimportant.

Signs

In adult breeding birds which are transmitting the organism to their progeny no signs of disease are visible. In infected poults there may be respiratory signs of coughing, sneezing, etc., but these are usually slight and in many infected flocks no such clinical signs are apparent. The main effect is reduced growth rate, poor food conversion and stunting. An occasional bird may show swelling of the facial sinuses, although this is much less prevalent than in *M.gallisepticum* infected flocks.

In the mid nineteen-sixties an increased incidence of leg problems was noted in turkey poults in England and America. The cause was at first unknown but it was eventually shown that there was an association between this condition and *M.meleagridis* infection. It is now believed that *M.meleagridis* is the main cause although the syndrome is similar to that seen in some cases of nutritional deficiency of factors such as manganese and choline. It is thought that the condition is the result of an interruption to the nutrient supply to the growth plates of certain long bones brought about by the mycoplasmal infection. Before the cause was known the condition was named "Turkey Syndrome '65" and this name is still sometimes used. The main features are shortening, bowing and twisting of the metatarsal bones (bones between the hocks and the feet), swelling of the hocks, stunting and poor feathering. The condition is usually first noticed in birds of two to four weeks of age, some of which make a partial recovery by eight weeks, while other more severely affected birds may have to be culled. A high incidence was common in the early days of the syndrome but at the present time, although a few cases may be seen in many flocks, an incidence of even 2 per cent is unusual. It should be emphasised that many *M.meleagridis* infected poults do not develop leg problems, but it is important to bear in mind that *M.meleagridis* can be responsible for a respiratory syndrome with reduced growth rate leading to stunting and also a form of leg abnormality. There are of course many leg weaknesses in turkeys which are unconnected with *M.meleagridis.*

Post Mortem Findings

The main change in uncomplicated *M.meleagridis* infection is airsacculitis or airsac disease. Affected air sacs are cloudy, thickened and have flecks of opaque pus adhering to their surfaces. Occasionally a swollen facial sinus with an accumulation of caseous material in the sinus cavity may be found.

Airsacculitis lesions are seen in poults from shortly after hatching up to sixteen weeks of age after which the lesions tend to regress and disappear unless complicated by *E.coli* or other bacterial infection. Where this is present it generally masks the milder changes produced by the underlying mycoplasmal infection.

The changes in the skeletal system already referred to will be confirmed at post mortem examination in cases of **turkey syndrome '65.**

Diagnosis

The clinical signs and post mortem changes in both the respiratory and skeletal syndromes are insufficient evidence on which to base a diagnosis although these may give rise to suspicion of the disease. Diagnosis depends on isolation of the causal agent in the laboratory (often a difficult procedure) or blood testing to show the presence of antibodies to the organism. A haemagglutination inhibition test or a rapid plate test may be used. It should be remembered however that in blood testing it is antibodies to the organism that are being demonstrated, and a positive blood test does not necessarily mean that the organism is involved in a disease process at the time the test is performed. This general principle should be borne in mind when blood testing for this or other infections.

Treatment

A number of antibiotics are available for treatment of *M.meleagridis* infection. These include **tylosin, erythromycin, spiramycin** and **spectinomycin.** Antibiotic therapy may be found more effective in some cases than in others; generally some beneficial effect results from treatment of poults, but antibiotic treatment of breeding birds in an attempt to prevent egg transmission of the disease gives disappointing results.

The antibiotics mentioned above are usually administered in the drinking water but some can also be given by injection.

Prevention and Control

Since *M.meleagridis* is essentially egg transmitted an effective method of prevention of this means of transmission should give a large measure of control of the disease. Most of the large turkey breeding organisations are now engaged in such control programmes which are made easier by the fact that transmission occurs by the transovarian route and that penetration of the egg shell by the organism after the egg is laid is not important. Hence methods of destroying organisms which are present within the egg when it is laid should give effective control of the disease. (This is in contrast to egg transmission of other diseases such as *E.coli* yolk sac infection or Aspergillosis in which penetration of the shell after the egg is laid is of major importance).

A number of methods of control of *M.meleagridis* have been investigated. As mentioned, drug treatment of the breeding bird has been tried, but is not effective. Since artificial insemination is now almost universally used in turkey breeding and since the disease is venereally spread between brooding birds, antibiotic treatment of semen might be expected to give control of the disease. This has been tried and has been successful in some cases although further investigation of the procedure is required.

The main methods of control involve treatment of the egg and are similar to those described for *M.gallisepticum* infection. Heat treatment of the egg is used but in the case of turkey eggs this often causes serious reduction in hatchability. Egg dipping in antibiotic solution using either temperature differential or pressure differential methods give good control. Tylosin or gentamicin solutions may be used, gentamicin being highly effective against mycoplasma and many species of bacteria.

Another technique used for control of *M.meleagridis* is injection of hatching eggs with antibiotic solution. This method is more certain than egg dipping as each egg receives a known dose of antibiotic. Tylosin or gentamicin solution is injected into the air cell of each egg between seven and fourteen days of incubation and it has been found that by this means transmission of the disease can be almost eliminated.

These egg treatments may be supplemented by other monitoring procedures such as blood testing and culturing of breeding birds to detect infection, followed by removal of such infected birds from breeding flocks. Culturing of dead-in-shell embryos, blood testing of poults hatching from treated eggs, and rearing of hatched poults in small groups are further useful measures in establishing infection free flocks. Eventual eradication of the disease by application of these various methods should be possible.

CHAPTER 14

Newcastle Disease

DEVELOPMENT

Newcastle Disease, one of the most important of all poultry diseases, takes its name from an outbreak which occurred near Newcastle-on-Tyne in 1927. It has since been identified in all the major poultry producing areas of the world and has been the cause of enormous financial loss to the poultry industries of many countries.

It appears that the virus of Newcastle Disease first infected poultry in Asia. Its spread was then facilitated by man, particularly in the form of transport of refrigerated meat which became an important industry about the time of the original outbreaks and by movement of human food waste containing remnants of poultry carcases.

In Britain the first outbreak at Newcastle was followed by several more in 1927. For several years after this the infection seemed to disappear, but in 1933 another outbreak was reported. The situation then remained quiescent until 1947 when a major epidemic took place, more than two thousand outbreaks occurring in that year. In view of the serious situation that had arisen, legislation was introduced to make the disease notifiable thus strengthening the slaughter and compensation policy previously introduced in 1936. The disease remains notifiable to the present time although the slaughter policy was discontinued in 1962.

New Virus

Outbreaks of the disease in Britain continued to occur more or less regularly. In 1950 it was shown that a milder form of the disease, prevalent earlier in America, was also present in Britain. This mild form of the disease became the one responsible for most outbreaks in Britain until 1970, when a sudden upsurge of the disease occurred due to a virus of increased virulence which spread with great rapidity. The strain was called "Essex 70" and it caused enormous loss to the industry before it was brought under control by increased use of vaccines and other measures. At present the disease incidence is very low, but there is a real danger of a virulent virus again gaining entry to the poultry population with devastating results. For this reason adequate vaccination of the national flock is essential.

CAUSE

Newcastle Disease is caused by a virus of the paramyxovirus group, of which many strains exist varying in virulence from very mild to extremely pathogenic. Strains also vary in their ability to attack various systems within the body. Some exert their effects mainly on the respiratory system, others on the nervous system. The virus has the ability to agglutinate or clump the red blood cells of chickens and various mammalian species, a property made use of in a blood test, the **haemagglutination inhibition test**, for detecting antibodies to the virus.

Animals susceptible

Natural infection with Newcastle Disease is usually restricted to chickens, turkeys and pheasants. Ducks, geese and pigeons are more resistant, although mild infections have been reported. The natural disease has also been recorded in various wild birds and others have been artificially infected. Exotic species such as parrots can also be infected. A mild form of the disease, in which conjunctivitis is a prominent sign, has occurred in humans.

SOURCE OF OUTBREAKS AND SPREAD OF DISEASE

Newcastle Disease virus may be introduced to a susceptible poultry population in a number of ways. These include purchase of stock replacements which are in the early stages of the disease, which have recently recovered from it, or which have been in contact with affected birds. Mechanical transmission of the virus on the hands, boots or clothing of visitors who have recently had contact with infected birds, and on poultry equipment such as crates, feed bags, egg cases and vehicles is a constant danger. Wild birds may transmit the disease, and airborne transmission from other nearby farms, will readily occur. The airborne route is the most important means of spread of the disease within a flock. The extreme contagiousness of the virus cannot be over-emphasised. Following infection of birds, rapid spread throughout the flock occurs. Virus is present in discharges and excreta from infected birds in high concentration, within two to four days of infection, and continues to be excreted for a number of weeks. A true carrier state, however, is not believed to exist. There is little evidence that egg transmission is an important means of spread although live virus has been found in eggs, and breakage of such eggs could act as a means of transmission of the disease.

In the frozen state the virus will live for many months, but at normal temperatures it will not survive for more than a few weeks. It is readily killed by most disinfectants used at the recommended strength.

SIGNS

Clinical signs of Newcastle Disease are extremely variable and depend on the virulence and dose of the infecting virus, the degree of immunity of the bird or flock, the age of the birds and various physical conditions such as temperature. In addition, some strains of virus produce mainly neurological signs and others mainly respiratory signs.

In general, at the start of an outbreak, birds may be noticed to be dull and quiet, with a tendency to stand around with ruffled feathers. Appetite is reduced. Where neurological signs predominate, leg and wing weakness may be seen together with muscular twitching, twisting of the neck and eventual paralysis with birds going off their legs and lying on their sides. These nervous signs may be accompanied by some respiratory difficulty and greenish diarrhoea. In other outbreaks nervous signs are less prominent and involvement of the respiratory system is the main syndrome. Generally, there is difficulty in breathing and other signs include gurgling, gasping and coughing. There may be a mucoid discharge from the eyes and nostrils and drooling of saliva from the mouth. Mortality rate may be high, but birds which survive for a few days often develop various nervous signs as described above, in particular twisting of the neck.

In **laying birds,** any of the above signs may occur accompanied by a sudden drop in egg production. In birds which have some immunity, or where a mild virus is involved, a production drop with soft shelled and shell-less eggs and loss of egg shell colour may be the only signs.

In **turkeys**, signs are similar to the respiratory signs in chickens but are generally less severe. Nervous signs are less common.

The variability of signs in Newcastle disease must again be emphasised. Also mortality may vary from zero to almost 100 per cent.

POST MORTEM FINDINGS

A number of well recognised pathological changes occur in Newcastle disease, but the severity of these varies depending on immunity, strain and virulence of infecting virus and other factors, as do clinical signs. The main changes are usually inflammation of the trachea, (tracheitis), haemorrhages in the fat of the heart and gizzard, haemorrhages in the proventriculus, cloudiness or frothiness of the air sacs and, in some cases, haemorrhages and ulceration of the intestines. All these changes, however, can be found in other diseases and are not diagnostic of Newcastle disease. In laying flocks, internal laying and egg peritonitis increase in incidence.

DIAGNOSIS

It must be emphasised that diagnosis of Newcastle disease is frequently not an easy matter. Where a number of cases have occurred in a country or geographical area further cases may be diagnosed with reasonable accuracy if typical signs and post mortem changes are present. Difficulties arise where such signs and pathological changes are slight or absent and in diagnosing, or even suspecting, an original outbreak in an area. However, in view of the importance of Newcastle disease, it should be at the forefront of the clinician's mind at all times. Diagnosis should in all cases be confirmed by isolation of the causative virus. For this, birds in the early stages of the disease should be submitted to a diagnostic laboratory. Virus can generally best be isolated from the trachea, but other tissues such as bone marrow and brain may on occasion yield virus readily. It is best to attempt isolation from several tissues in order to increase the likelihood of success. Actual isolation is made by injecting an extract of these tissues into the allantoic sac of embryonated eggs derived from a disease free flock. Further tests are then performed to identify the virus.

A blood test, known as **haemagglutination inhibition test,** may also be used as an aid to diagnosis of the disease. The basis of the test is that Newcastle disease virus when mixed with a suspension of chicken red blood cells, causes them to clump together or agglutinate, and that birds which have encountered the virus develop antibodies in their blood serum which neutralise the virus and prevent it from agglutinating red blood cells. To perform the test, blood serum from a number of birds involved in a suspected Newcastle disease outbreak is mixed with Newcastle disease virus and red blood cells added. Antibodies in sera from infected birds neutralise the virus and red blood cells are not agglutinated. The sera of non-infected birds does not contain antibodies, the virus is not neutralised and the red cells are agglutinated. This test is of considerable value as it is rapid, simple to perform and inexpensive, but it suffers from the disadvantage that in Britain and other countries where vaccination against Newcastle disease is performed, this procedure also causes the production of haemagglutination-inhibiting antibodies and it is frequently impossible to differentiate between a positive test due to infection by field virus or infection by vaccine virus. This is particularly the case where a field virus of low virulence may be involved as the titre, or degree to which the test is positive, due to such a virus will be similar to the titre due to vaccinal virus.

A further diagnostic procedure sometimes used is histological examination of the trachea, which in most cases will at least differentiate the disease from acute infectious bronchitis. Again, however, the issue may be complicated by the fact that similar, though milder changes are produced by live virus vaccination.

Diagnosis may be further complicated by the presence of other disease in a flock along with Newcastle disease. For example colisepticaemia commonly occurs in broiler flocks and is readily diagnosed, but the possibility of an underlying Newcastle disease infection being masked by the more obvious secondary bacterial infection should be borne in mind. In all cases where respiratory or nervous signs occur in a flock Newcastle disease should be considered as a possible cause.

TREATMENT

There is no effective treatment for Newcastle disease. Antibiotics have no effect on the virus although they may help to control secondary infection. In countries where vaccination is used, immediate spray vaccination of a flock with live virus vaccine in the earliest stages of an outbreak may give a measure of control if the vaccine virus can establish itself in the flock before the field virus has had time to spread throughout the flock. However, bearing in mind the very rapid spread of field virus within a flock, the value of this procedure must in most cases be considered doubtful.

PREVENTION AND CONTROL

There are two main methods of combating Newcastle Disease in addition to efficient hygiene methods. These are control by slaughter of infected flocks and prevention by vaccination.

The slaughter policy was used in Britain until the early nineteen sixties. When infection occurred in a flock all birds on the premises were slaughtered and their bodies burned or buried. Compensation was paid to the owner. The aim in a slaughter policy is to eliminate the virus as rapidly and effectively as possible and so prevent spread to other flocks. It is still used in some countries, but in Britain, for various reasons, was abandoned in 1962 and a vaccination policy introduced.

Two main types of vaccines are now used in Britain. These are **live virus vaccines** and **inactivated** (or killed) **vaccines.** Live vaccines are further known as **Hitchener B1** the milder strain, and **La Sota** the stronger type. Generally, live vaccines are administered at intervals during rearing and a single dose of inactivated vaccine given at point of lay. In broilers only live vaccines are used, while in turkeys inactivated vaccines are generally used due to their greater effectiveness in this species, although live vaccines may also be used.

Live vaccines may be administered in the drinking water, by aerosol spray or by eye-drop. Each method has advantages and disadvantages; for example, drinking water vaccination is easily carried out but is least effective, whereas spray vaccination is more effective but requires an aerosol generator for its application and is more likely to give rise to post-vaccinal respiratory symptoms in the birds, which may be followed by secondary bacterial infection and some mortality. The eye-drop method is effective and ensures that every bird is individually dosed, but this entails handling all birds in the flock, which is impractical where very large numbers are involved.

Inactivated vaccines give rise to considerably higher antibody levels than live vaccines, but, again, since they are given by injection, all birds must be handled. However this is conveniently done in the case of laying flocks at the time of moving the birds from their rearing to their laying quarters when they are handled in any case. An injection of inactivated vaccine at this time will protect birds through their laying year, whereas if inactivated vaccines are not used it may be necessary to re-vaccinate with live vaccine at intervals during lay.

Various vaccination programmes are used and some guidance is given in the manufacturer's instruction leaflets which accompany the vaccine.

It should be understood that live vaccines act by infecting the birds and giving rise to a mild attack of the disease which stimulates immunity. Inactivated vaccines, on the other hand, contain killed virus. They require to be injected and, being oil-based, are retained at the injection site for some time, giving rise to prolonged stimulation of the bird's immunological system and hence high levels of immunity.

It is possible to assess the flock's immune state following vaccination by measuring the level of haemagglutination inhibiting antibodies in sera of blood samples taken from a number of birds in the flock. The titre or level of these antibodies will give some indication of the efficiency of a vaccination programme. A number of diagnostic laboratories are able to undertake this work and many flocks are routinely blood tested in this way.

Finally it must again be mentioned that Newcastle disease is notifiable and the Divisional Veterinary Office of the Ministry of Agriculture should be informed when the disease is diagnosed or suspected.

CHAPTER 15

Infectious Bronchitis

NATURE OF DISEASE

Infectious bronchitis is an acute, highly contagious respiratory disease of poultry caused by a virus, the most severe clinical effects of which are seen in young chicks but which also causes serious economic losses due to drops in egg production when it affects laying birds.

Following the first report of the disease in America in 1931 it was soon found to be prevalent in many parts of that country, particularly where birds were reared intensively. It is still an important cause of financial loss in many parts of the world including Britain, although it has been partly controlled by use of vaccination. It was first shown to exist in Britain in 1948, during work on Newcastle disease when it was found that a respiratory syndrome of a milder type than the virulent form of Newcastle disease then prevalent, was not Newcastle disease but a completely separate disease, infectious bronchitis.

CAUSE

Infectious bronchitis is caused by a virus of the *Coronavirus* group. The virus will survive for several months at refrigerator temperature but is usually killed within fourteen days at room temperature. It is also killed quite easily by most commonly used disinfectants.

INCIDENCE IN BRITAIN

The exact incidence of the disease in Britain is difficult to assess accurately, particularly since the advent of live virus vaccines. These have been highly effective in controlling the main signs of the disease but have made the task of the diagnostician more difficult in that their effects tend to simulate those of a mild disease outbreak. Also, exact diagnosis of infectious bronchitis and its differentiation from other respiratory diseases can be time consuming and expensive so that some milder outbreaks may remain undiagnosed. In addition some outbreaks of respiratory disease may well commence as infectious bronchitis, but other pathogens, notably *Escherichia coli*, become superimposed and mask the primary infection. There is no doubt that the incidence of respiratory disease generally has increased in step with intensivism in the industry, the infectious bronchitis virus being one of the prime pathogens involved in the respiratory disease complex.

Under natural conditions, infectious bronchitis occurs in chickens only; other domesticated birds including turkeys are unaffected.

SOURCE OF OUTBREAKS

The virus of infectious bronchitis may be introduced to a susceptible flock by airborne spread, by contaminated equipment, including vehicles, or by buying in of infected or carrier birds. The recovered carrier state, however, probably does not persist for more than about two months following infection. Airborne tranmission may well be the most important means of dissemination of the virus in a neighbourhood. There is no evidence for the occurrence of vertical transmission of the virus from dam to offspring via the egg.

Once infection has been introduced to a susceptible flock the virus spreads rapidly throughout the flock and to other flocks on the premises. The incubation period is short, signs usually developing within thirty-six to forty-eight hours of infection. This, however, will depend on the strain and virulence of virus involved.

SIGNS

The signs produced by infectious bronchitis virus in a flock depend on the age of bird involved. The most severe clinical signs occur in young chicks and consist of gasping, coughing and noisy breathing. There may be a discharge from the eyes and nostrils. The chicks become depressed and lethargic and tend to huddle under the brooder. Appetite and growth rate are reduced. Mortality in young chicks may be 25 per cent but this depends on the strain of virus, the general health of the flock and the level of parental antibody present in the chicks.

The main signs of infectious bronchitis in older chicks and growers are some disturbance in breathing, general inactivity and loss of appetite. Retarded growth will result, which is more noticeable and of more significance in broilers than in pullet chicks.

In birds over a few weeks of age, mortality in the uncomplicated disease is slight but it must be emphasised that, particularly in broilers, bronchitis infection is frequently followed by invasion of the respiratory system by *Escherichia coli*, giving rise to **colisepticaemia**. This secondary bacterial infection can be much more important than the viral infection which gave rise to it.

Effect on egg-laying

An effect of infectious bronchitis virus infection which is sometimes overlooked is that in **baby chicks** the virus may attack the oviduct with the result that when these birds reach laying age, they fail to come into production because of developmental abnormalities of the oviduct. If there is a significant number of these non-producers, production targets may not be achieved.

In **laying birds** the main effects of bronchitis virus infection are not in the respiratory system in which signs are usually slight or absent, but on the egg-laying mechanism. There is a drop in production of up to 50 per cent, depending on the virulence of the virus, the resistance of the birds and the period of lay. Older flocks usually suffer a greater drop than younger flocks. Following infection in laying birds, recovery is usually slow and incomplete, the production graph becoming irregular and failing to return to pre-infection level. There is also serious loss of egg quality, shells becoming rough, ridged and mis-shapen, and albumen becoming thinner than normal, a condition often referred to as "watery-white". These egg changes may persist to some degree for the rest of the life of the flock.

Kidney disease

In Australia there occurs a strain of infectious brochitis virus known as the **"T" strain.** This particular virus attacks the bird's kidneys causing a condition known in Australia as **Cummings Disease**. A similar condition occurs in Britain and recent research suggests that strains other than the known nephrotoxic "T" strain

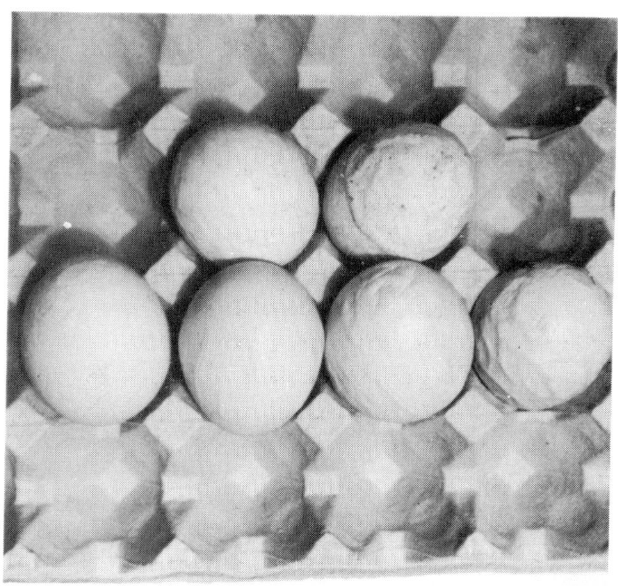

15.1 Eggs from flock which had experienced infectious bronchitis outbreak during lay. Note the ridged and wrinkled shells.

may be involved. Further work is required to establish the precise role of infectious bronchitis virus strains in avian kidney disease.

POST MORTEM FINDINGS AND DIAGNOSIS

In chicks which die of the disease or which are killed while affected, there is excess mucus in the trachea and the nasal passages and sinuses. Grossly visible inflammation of the trachea is usually not marked, although there may be slight reddening of the upper trachea and larynx. This change is certainly not as distinct as in the more severe forms of Newcastle disease or Infectious Laryngotracheitis. There may be mild pneumonic change in the lungs and cloudiness of the air sacs.

These changes generally become less evident with increasing age of affected birds and in adult layers changes in the respiratory system are slight or absent. There may however be visible decrease in oviduct length, and fluid egg yolk material may be found in the abdominal cavity. The effects on eggs produced in the course of the disease and following recovery in some birds have already been described.

91

Lesions of the oviduct may be found in birds of laying age which survived an infectious bronchitis outbreak in early life. Parts of the oviduct show developmental abnormalities, the middle part in some cases being almost entirely absent.

In birds infected by the "T" strain or other nephrotoxic strains the kidneys show varying degrees of swelling and paleness, and the ureters (tubes which convey urine from the kidneys to the cloaca) become greatly distended with white urate deposits.

Neither clinical signs nor grossly visible changes due to infectious bronchitis are sufficiently characteristic to distinguish the disease from other respiratory infections and in order to establish a diagnosis further laboratory tests are necessary. In severe acute cases histological examination of the trachea reveals a rather typical microscopic picture which may be sufficient to confirm a diagnosis. In milder cases however these changes may be less marked and it should be borne in mind that similar changes will result from use of live virus vaccination. This must be taken into account by diagnosticians in flocks where such vaccines are in use. Other tests involve the demonstration of neutralising or precipitating antibodies in blood serum and isolation of the causative virus. Absolute diagnosis of the disease, its differentiation from other respiratory conditions and elucidation of the part it plays in the respiratory disease complex in any particular instance can present the clinician with considerable problems.

TREATMENT, PREVENTION AND CONTROL

No treatment has any appreciable effect on the causative virus. However provision of adequate ventilation, avoidance of overcrowding, maintenance of feed intake and other anti-stress measures will aid recovery. The use of antibiotics to prevent secondary bacterial infection may be justified but it should be clearly understood that these have no effect on the virus itself.

Management procedures such as isolation of flocks and adoption of "all-in, all-out" rearing systems wherever practicable will help to prevent the disease, but outbreaks can still occur in spite of all precautions. Therefore, it was deemed necessary to attempt to prevent the disease by vaccination and vaccines against the disease have now been available in Britain for a number of years. These are **live virus vaccines** and the strains most commonly used are referred to as **"H120"** (weak, 1B1) and **"H52"** (strong, 1B2). As a general rule in the case of future laying birds, the "H120" vaccine is administered at approximately three weeks of age and the "H52" at approximately fourteen weeks of age and in the case of broilers a single "H120" is given at two to three weeks. However, vaccination programmes are many and varied, and may be modified to suit the particular needs and circumstances of each individual producer.

It should be said that use of live vaccines is equivalent to giving the flock a mild dose of the disease concerned. This necessarily involves some degree of respiratory stress, which may be followed by bacterial infection of the respiratory system and, in some cases, significant mortality, particularly in broilers. For this reason some broiler growers prefer to avoid the use of live vaccines, but by failing to vaccinate they leave their stock open to challenge by virulent field virus.

Live vaccines may be administered either in the drinking water or by aerosol spray. The latter method generally stimulates greater immune response but may give rise to more respiratory stress in the birds. The manufacturers' instructions for use and storage should be carefully observed if the maximum effect is to be achieved.

In the case of pullet flocks it is useful to monitor response to vaccination by measurement of antibody levels in blood sera of a sample of birds from the flock. This should be done before point-of-lay but after the vaccination programme has been completed. Should the antibody levels be considered insufficient to protect the flock through lay a further vaccination may be given before the birds come into production.

CHAPTER 16

Infectious Laryngotracheitis

NATURE AND INCIDENCE

Infectious laryngotracheitis (I.L.T.) is another of the group of important viral respiratory diseases of poultry. It occurs in chickens and pheasants only, other birds being resistant to natural and, in most cases, to experimental infection. It generally affects adult poultry, but birds of all ages are susceptible.

The disease was first reported in America in 1925 and was soon shown to be fairly widely distributed in that country. It is still a considerable threat to the industry in some areas of America although vaccination has helped to bring it under control. In Britain it now occurs mainly in a number of distinct areas, e.g. in and around Lancashire, although in other parts of the country sporadic outbreaks can occur at any time.

CAUSE

The disease is caused by a virus of the herpes group. The virus is easily killed by commonly available disinfectants and by direct sunlight, although it can survive for considerable periods of time in the frozen state.

SOURCE OF OUTBREAKS AND SPREAD OF THE DISEASE

In areas where the disease is still fairly common, probably the main source of outbreaks is the symptomless carrier bird. The virus can be isolated from tissues of these recovered birds for very long periods and transmission from carriers to susceptible birds following mixing or contact will readily occur. Once present, carriers may perpetuate the infection in a flock from year to year until complete depopulation can be arranged.

It is also possible that the virus may be introduced by contaminated crates and equipment, or by persons who have recently visited other premises during an outbreak. These indirect methods of spread, and airborne infection, are less important in the case of infectious laryngotracheitis than in Newcastle disease and infectious bronchitis; **spread by carrier birds** is undoubtedly most important. Egg transmission of I.L.T. virus has not been shown to occur.

When the disease occurs in a flock, it spreads fairly rapidly but not as fast as Newcastle disease or infectious bronchitis. Also, unlike the latter diseases, it may be possible to prevent flock to flock spread for a prolonged period where flocks are fairly well separated and where hygienic standards are high, even without the use of vaccination. However, as will be mentioned later, immediate vaccination of neighbouring flocks would be advisable in the event of an outbreak.

Signs

The incubation period of I.L.T. virus is about seven to ten days. The first sign of the disease is usually a watery discharge from the eyes and nostrils followed rapidly by difficulty in breathing, gurgling and rattling noises, coughing and gasping. Affected birds tend to sit on their hocks with their necks extended and beaks wide open during inspiration which may be accompanied by a high-pitched whistling sound. They shake their heads as though attempting to remove an obstruction from the trachea. Their efforts frequently terminate in the coughing up of blood clots or blood-stained mucus which gives them some temporary relief from their respiratory distress. In some cases so much blood may be coughed up that it is readily noticed on the floor and walls of the cages or poulty-house.

The above description is of a severe form of I.L.T. in which mortality may reach 20 per cent, deaths in many birds occurring within two or three days of the onset of symptoms. In milder or more chronic forms of I.L.T., mortality rate may be only 2 per cent or less with much less severe respiratory signs, perhaps only watery eyes, nasal discharge and slight coughing, but these effects may persist in the flock for up to several months.

In the severe form of the disease there is a considerable drop in egg production, although in many cases production loss is less than in Newcastle disease and infectious bronchitis. Surviving birds usually return to normal egg production within three weeks of first showing signs of the disease but they may continue to harbour the virus and eliminate it intermittently for as long as two years.

Post Mortem Findings and Diagnosis

Post mortem changes are confined to the respiratory tract. In severe cases there is extremely acute inflammation of the trachea, the lining or mucus membrane of the entire upper trachea and larynx becoming bright red in appearance with haemorrhages in the mucous membrane; in some cases, free blood or a mixture of blood and mucus may partially obstruct the tracheal lumen. In cases which have survived for several days, the lining of the trachea undergoes necrosis or death of tissue, becoming greenish-yellow in colour and partially detached from the underlying tissue. As mucus adheres to this dead tissue and dries up, the larynx or trachea may be completely obstructed by a caseous necrotic mass and the bird dies of asphyxiation.

The changes described above are typical of severe I.L.T. and are unlikely to occur in any other disease. In less severe cases, however the post mortem findings are much less typical consisting of mild tracheitis with mucus in the tracheal lumen. There may or may not be some haemorrhages in the mucous membrane. There is often conjunctivitis and inflammatory reaction of the nasal mucous membrane and sinuses. Caseous deposits may be present under the eyelids. These changes are not sufficiently distinctive to distinguish the disease from other respiratory infections and in these cases further diagnostic procedures are required to establish a diagnosis. These may include blood tests for precipitating antibodies to the virus, histological examination of tracheas and isolation of the virus by injection of a suspension of tracheal or lung tissue into embryonating chicken eggs. Live birds should be submitted to a diagnostic laboratory when these tests are required.

Treatment

No drugs are of any value in treating the disease. In the event of an outbreak, vaccination of all unaffected birds should be performed as rapidly as possible. As the virus tends to spread less rapidly than other respiratory diseases this procedure can save many birds.

PREVENTION AND CONTROL

As with any infectious disease, hygiene measures are important in preventing introduction of infection from external sources. Following an outbreak, the danger of the infection being retained on the premises by recovered carrier birds must be borne in mind and all stock introduced must be vaccinated against the disease. This policy of vaccination should be maintained until such time as a complete "disease break" can be arranged.

In areas where the disease is endemic, vaccination of all stock should be practised. In areas where the disease is not common, vaccination is generally considered unnecessary; but it must be remembered that sporadic outbreaks can occur anywhere at any time and any delay in obtaining vaccine at the moment it is required may allow a spread to other flocks to occur in the meantime.

Vaccination of pullets where required is generally performed at eight to fourteen weeks of age. The vaccine, a live attenuated strain of I.L.T. virus, is applied by eye-drop to each bird individually. Where this is not possible it may be administered in the drinking water but this method gives less reliable results and may leave part of the flock with inadequate protection. Spray vaccination is also used, but can only be recommended where rapid results are required in the face of an outbreak, as it gives rise to a severe reaction in the birds and may result in significant mortality.

CHAPTER 17

Avian Encephalomyelitis

NATURE AND INCIDENCE

Avian encephalomyelitis or epidemic tremor as it is commonly named, is a viral infection which causes primarily a condition of the central nervous system in young chicks. In addition, when the infection occurs in a laying flock, it causes a sharp drop in egg production. Although at present it is not a major cause of loss to the industry generally in Britain, it can be a significant problem to the individual on whose premises it occurs and particularly to breeding organisations when breeding flocks are affected.

The first outbreak reported was in America in 1930. Other cases followed quickly with increasing incidence until the disease was found in most parts of the American continent. Since then it has been recognised in many parts of the world. Publication of its occurrence in Britain did not appear until 1955 since when the incidence increased for a number of years until control by vaccination became standard procedure, particularly in breeding flocks. At the present time outbreaks of avian encephalomyelitis in young chicks is not common but sporadic cases still occur.

The disease is seen mainly in chickens although pheasants and quail are said to be affected on rare occasions. There is no seasonal incidence and chickens of any breed may be affected.

Spread of Infection

Soon after avian encephalomyelitis was first reported it was shown to be infectious and to be caused by a virus. For many years the exact method of spread was not understood but it is now known that the virus is egg-transmitted. This implies that, following infection of a susceptible breeding flock, the virus is carried in the blood stream to the ovaries, enters the developing ova and is thus passed through the egg to infect the embryo. When the egg hatches the disease becomes manifest in the chick and the chick then eliminates the virus in its droppings, spreading the infection to its companions. It is believed that in many cases, only a small number of chicks may be infected via the egg, the main mode of dissemination of the virus being lateral spread from these chicks to their flock-mates.

The source and means of spread of the virus to growing or adult flocks, either breeders or commercial layers, is still uncertain but it is believed that direct or indirect mechanical transmission, such as in infected faeces, feed, water, is important. It appears that these birds must swallow the virus to become infected. Experiments to transmit the virus by aerosol have failed.

SIGNS

The name epidemic tremor refers to a trembling of the head and neck which is apparent in some cases. This tremor, however, in many cases is only slight and intermittent and may not be noticed unless chicks are observed very carefully. Certainly the signs of imbalance are usually more obvious.

The signs shown by birds infected by the encephalomyelitis virus depend on the age at which infection occurs. There are three distinct age groups, infection of which results in different clinical syndromes. Baby chicks show nervous signs, growing birds show no visible evidence of disease and flocks in lay suffer a drop in egg production, but again without visible clinical signs.

In **baby chicks** infected by egg transmission, signs are mainly associated with malfunction of the cerebellum, that part of the brain which controls balance. Chicks may be affected at hatching, but frequently in such small numbers that they are not noticed. These chicks pass the infection to their companions with the result that signs usually become apparent at one to two weeks of age. Some dullness and apathy may be noticed to begin with and a little later the chicks appear to lose proper control of balance so that they stumble about in a "drunken" manner. This imbalance becomes more obvious if the chicks are moved around or excited. Eventually they collapse on their haunches or fall over on their sides. Some refuse to move and emit weakened cries. In the later stages, affected chicks are incapable of moving, they fail to find food or water, and prostration and death soon follow. Affected chicks are often trampled upon by their pen-mates.

Care of affected chicks

It is possible by careful "nursing", separation of affected chicks and by making food and water easily available, to keep some chicks alive so that they eventually recover from the disease. It is unlikely that such recovered chicks would become useful production units whether for meat or egg production and under commercial conditions there is little point in keeping affected birds alive.

The mortality level in outbreaks of encephalomyelitis is very variable. In some cases it is less than 5 per cent, in others it may be 25 per cent.

Signs in older birds

When encephalomyelitis occurs in birds between three to four weeks and point of lay, no visible clinical signs are seen but a solid immunity is produced which protects the flock against the disease throughout lay. Where infection occurs in a non-immune laying flock a sudden considerable drop in egg production will occur. This production drop may be 25 per cent or more, but it is usually of short duration, the flock returning to normal production within about two weeks. Again no clinical signs are shown by the birds and it must be emphasised that infections occurring in birds of more than three to four weeks of age do not give rise to nervous signs such as are seen in infected baby chicks.

Post Mortem Findings and Diagnosis

No significant grossly visible pathological changes have been found in birds of any age which have suffered an encephalomyelitis infection. Histological examination of various organs including brain, spinal cord, pancreas and proventriculus from young chicks shows changes which are characteristic of the disease; in order to confirm a diagnosis, live affected chicks should be submitted to a laboratory suitably equipped to undertake this work. It is usually necessary to have this examination performed in order to differentiate the disease from others, including Vitamin E deficiency (crazy chick disease) and Newcastle disease in which nervous signs are also prominent.

In adult birds, even histological changes are slight or absent, making confirmation of diagnosis in these birds extremely difficult. However a **blood test** exists which is sometimes used in confirmation of diagnosis. A strongly positive test following a sharp drop in production in a laying flock for which no other explanation is apparent, is strongly suggestive of avian encephalomyelitis.

TREATMENT, PREVENTION AND CONTROL

There is no treatment of any value for avian encephalomyelitis. It is best to cull all affected chicks. In the case of adult birds, again no treatment is available, but additional vitamins supplied via the drinking water may help to restore egg production.

The disease can be **prevented by vaccination** of breeding or commercial laying stock with a live virus vaccine administered in the drinking water between the ages of ten and eighteen weeks. In commercial layers production drops are prevented and in breeders, in addition immunity is transferred through the egg to the progeny, giving these protection for the first eight weeks or so of life.

Response to vaccination can be assessed either by use of the blood test mentioned earlier, which measures response to vaccine virus as well as field virus, or in breeding flocks by means of a test known as the **embryo susceptibility test.** For this test fertile eggs are required. These are incubated for six days and the embryos are then injected with a measured amount of encephalomyelitis virus. Following a further six days of incubation the eggs are broken and the embryos examined for certain lesions; an assessment is made of the immune state of the parent flock from the number of embryos showing these lesions. In immune flocks, antibodies are passed to the embryos so that they are protected from the virus, whereas non-immune flocks provide no antibody protection and the embryos succumb to the virus.

Vaccination of all breeding stock should, in theory, totally prevent outbreaks of the disease in young chicks, and, indeed, the incidence of the disease has been greatly reduced. Occasional outbreaks still occur, however, possibly due to inadequate vaccination of breeding stock which are therefore at risk when a field challenge occurs. It is important to ensure that vaccination is properly and efficiently carried out at the correct age with vaccine which has been correctly stored and is fully potent.

CHAPTER 18

Infectious Bursal Disease

NATURE AND INCIDENCE

Infectious bursal disease is a virus disease of chickens which was first recorded near the small town of Gumboro in the U.S.A. in 1957, from which it takes its common name of **Gumboro disease**. It first affected the broiler population almost exclusively, but now occurs also in pullet flocks.

The disease is of considerable economic importance both from the point of view of clinical disease and mortality, as occurs in some infected flocks, and also because of the ability of the virus to cause a suppression of the bird's immune mechanisms, an effect which can occur even in completely subclinical infections. The result of this immuno-suppression is a lack of antibody production and a lowered resistance of affected birds to other disease-causing agents. Present day research into infectious bursal disease is concerned mainly with this immuno-suppressive effect.

Since its first occurrence in America, the disease has spread to the extent that it has been recorded in almost all important poultry rearing areas of the world. There has been a good deal of speculation concerning the reasons for the sudden appearance of this apparently new virus but no theory as to the origin and establishment of the virus in the poultry population has yet received universal acceptance.

CAUSE

For some time after its appearance the cause of the disease was in doubt. It was confused with a type of infectious bronchitis virus infection which involves the kidneys and in which the post mortem changes resemble those of infectious bursal disease. Eventually, however, the diseases were differentiated and the causal agent of infectious bursal disease was recognised as a separate virus, which was named **infectious bursal agent** because of its effects on the cloacal bursa.

Although the viral nature of the disease is now well known, the virus has so far eluded the attempts of virologists to classify it. At various times it has been associated with reoviruses and picornaviruses but it appears that at present it cannot be placed in any of the established viral groups.

Many strains of infectious bursal disease virus of varying virulence exist. This variation is mainly responsible for the widely different degrees of clinical involvement in affected flocks. In some cases the disease is totally subclinical; in others there are several clinical signs and high mortality. The virus is also noted for its high degree of stability and its resistance to environmental influences and to many of the commonly used disinfectants.

Occurrence

As already mentioned, infectious bursal disease occurs on a world-wide scale. It is seen most commonly in broilers of two to six weeks but also occurs in pullets. It has in fact been recorded in birds up to fifteen weeks of age. It does not occur in turkeys or other domestic species.

Although clinical disease is now less commonly seen than a few years ago, there is evidence that subclinical infection is widespread in Britain and Europe. The reduction in clinical disease may be associated with the recent introduction of a vaccination policy in a number of countries including the U.K. In some areas of the world where particularly virulent virus exists, vaccination has not given adequate control and severe disease still occurs.

Spread

The virus is shed in the droppings of infected birds resulting in heavy contamination of the environment and rapid spread within the flock. Spread between flocks, or even between pens in a house, however, is less rapid and probably depends on mechanical transmission of the virus by attendants or by contaminated feed or water. Air-borne spread has not been conclusively demonstrated.

There is evidence that meal-worms or other insect inhabitants of poultry houses may act as vectors of the virus. Egg transmission, while not totally excluded, appears not to be important and there is little evidence for the existence of recovered carrier birds.

It is a feature of infectious bursal disease that once introduced to a farm it tends to become endemic and persist from crop to crop even if depopulation is practised. The severity of disease however may vary from one crop to the next and an occasional crop may escape infection completely. In some cases the diseases may remain localised to one part of a house and may apparently clear up only to reappear in another part of the house some days later. These characteristics of the disease are doubtless due largely to the resistance of the virus and to the mainly mechanical means of transmission.

SIGNS

Affected birds show general depression and loss of appetite. They stand apart from their flock-mates and are reluctant to move. In some birds there may be signs of trembling or unsteady gait. There may also be evidence of vent pecking and watery white diarrhoea. Growth rate is slowed and time to market may be significantly increased.

The duration of illness is short and very sick birds seldom recover. Mortality rises sharply to a peak and also declines sharply. Individual birds generally die or recover in four or five days and recovery of the flock (or part of it) is usually complete in two weeks from the onset of signs. Losses are usually 5 to 10 per cent but in severe outbreaks may reach 30 per cent. Generally, the older the flock at the start of an outbreak, the lower the mortality.

Post Mortem Findings

There are a number of well-defined pathological changes associated with infectious bursal disease. It should be stressed however that not all these changes are seen in every carcase, and in some mild outbreaks changes are almost undetectable. Hence, in some outbreaks, diagnosis may be made quite accurately from post mortem findings alone, while in other cases this is not possible and additional procedures are necessary.

In many birds multiple haemorrhages occur in the thigh and breast muscles and are easily visible on removing the skin. These haemorrhages, which tend to be elongated and lie along the line of the muscle fibres, are rather characteristic and are seen in few diseases other than infectious bursal disease. Haemorrhages also occur in the mucosa of the proventriculus, in many cases in a narrow zone at the junction of the proventriculus and gizzard. Also visible on opening the carcase are changes in the kidneys: these are usually pale and swollen, with tubules distended by urates; urates may also fill the ureters.

The most characteristic changes in infections bursal disease, however, occur in the cloacal bursa. This is a small, hollow, approximately spherical organ attached to the upper wall of the rectum immediately inside the cloaca. In affected birds it is enlarged, turgid and its normal creamy-white colour may be changed to pale pink or dark red or any intermediate colour. In addition, the bursa may be oedematous, and in some cases a caseous deposit will be found inside the bursa, its shape reflecting the folded interior of the organ. These bursal changes are quite specific for infectious bursal disease and are unlikely to be seen in any other condition.

Other occasional changes which may be seen in the disease are slight swelling and paleness of the liver, enlargement of the spleen and dehydration of the carcase.

Diagnosis

It has already been mentioned that in outbreaks of infectious bursal disease in which typical signs and post mortem changes are present, a diagnosis may be made without further investigation. In many cases, however, these signs and changes are not sufficient evidence on which to base a diagnosis. In these cases, the most reliable means of confirming a diagnosis is by histological examination of the cloacal bursa. Microscopic examination of sections of affected bursae show characteristic degenerative changes which occur only in infectious bursal disease. These changes are not produced by vaccine strains of the virus so that diagnosis is not complicated by vaccination.

Virus isolation is also sometimes used to confirm diagnosis. This may be done in embryonating eggs or by tissue culture methods. Obviously, where these procedures are required, birds must be submitted to a well equipped laboratory.

TREATMENT AND CONTROL

There is no specific treatment for infectious bursal disease. Antibiotics and other drugs have no effect on the virus.

Following an outbreak complete removal of old litter and disinfection of the premises, preferably with an iodophor type of disinfectant, followed by fumigation are essential measures. Complete destruction of the virus, however, proves impossible in many cases.

Live virus vaccines have been used in some countries for a number of years. These, however, have been considered unsuitable for use in Britain for various reasons and only recently has a vaccine suitable for use in this country been developed. The vaccine is administered to breeding stock and maternal antibodies transferred to the chicks protect these for the first two to three weeks. Various additional vaccination regimes for broilers have been suggested. Where parents have been adequately vaccinated with sufficient transfer of antibody, a single vaccination at thirty days is normally recommended. If parents are not vaccinated, vaccination of progeny at day old and again at fourteen days and thirty days may be necessary.

INFECTIOUS BURSAL DISEASE AND IMMUNO-SUPPRESSION

It was mentioned earlier that the infectious bursal agent is of importance not only because of the clinical syndrome and mortality which may result from infection of a susceptible flock, but also because of the effect of the virus on the chick's immune system in early life. The virus principally affects the cloacal bursa, spleen and thymus, organs which play a major part in the development of the immune response, especially circulating antibody production, in the young chick. Infection of the bursa by the virus in the first two weeks of life results in a form of bursal degeneration which seriously reduces the chick's ability to form antibodies to, and thereby resist, other infectious agents. It has been shown that early infection by infectious bursal disease virus results in higher mortality from *E.coli* and *Salmonella typhimurium* as well increasing the flock's susceptibility to inclusion body hepatitis and gangrenous dermatitis.

Another important consequence of the effect of the virus on the bird's immune system is that immunological response to administration of vaccines, including those against Newcastle disease, infectious bronchitis, Marek's disease and fowl pox, may be reduced, resulting in less than optimal protection against these diseases following vaccination. This may explain some of the disappointing antibody titres commonly found on blood testing for the purpose of monitoring immune response. Vaccination of parent flocks against infectious bursal disease with transference of maternal antibody to the progeny should help to prevent infectious bursal disease in young chicks and overcome associated immunologocial problems.

CHAPTER 19

Fowl Pox

NATURE AND INCIDENCE

Fowl pox is an infectious disease of poulty associated typically with the presence of wart-like eruptions on the comb and wattles. It has been known since time immemorial and has caused considerable loss to the poultry industry throughout the world.

Pox occurs wherever poultry are raised but its distribution is not regular. It may be extremely common in one part of a country and rare in another. For example in Britain, Lancashire has had considerable trouble, but in many other areas it is almost unheard of. Once pox becomes established on a farm it is difficult to eradicate and may recur from year to year.

Fowl pox virus affects chickens, but closely related strains of virus also affect pigeons, turkeys and canaries. Ducks and geese are only rarely affected. Breeds of chicks having large combs, such as Leghorns are considered to be most susceptible.

CAUSE

Fowl pox was one of the first diseases shown to be caused by a virus and, as such, it has been intensively studied. Unlike bacteria, viruses can only multiply within the cells of the animal affected, the particular cells involved in pox infection being principally those of the unfeathered regions of the skin and the mucous membranes lining the mouth and throat.

In general, viruses are not visible under the ordinary light microscope because of their extremely small size. Pox viruses, however, become aggregated together in the infected cells and the aggregations, or inclusion bodies, are sufficiently large to be seen under the microscope. Each inclusion body may consist of up to 20,000 virus particles, each capable of setting up the disease in a susceptible bird.

The causal virus is extremely resistant to drying and survives for long periods, up to twelve months or even more, under varying climatic conditions. A pox scab removed from a wild turkey and stored in a refrigerator was found to contain viable virus eight years later. On the other hand, it is destroyed fairly rapidly by moist heat and by most disinfectants. It is, however, extremely resistant to the action of some agents such as glycerine, which destroy bacteria. Glycerine, in fact, is sometimes used as a preservative for pox virus preparations.

Four different forms of pox are recognised and are named according to the species normally affected, that is to say: **fowl pox, turkey pox, pigeon pox and canary pox.** In general, the virus strains infecting each species will also infect others but the disease they cause in these other species is usually mild and transient. Infection by one virus strain confers solid immunity against future infection with the same strain. It may also confer immunity, which is usually less complete, against infection by other strains.

Transmission

The fowl pox virus is unable to infect unbroken skin or mucous membrane and infection usually occurs through cuts, scratches or abrasions on the comb, wattles, other unfeathered skin regions and in the mouth. These injuries may be the result of fighting and pecking. Infection of a clean flock will readily result from mechanical transmission of the virus by persons, vehicles or equipment. In some countries the disease is spread by mosquitoes. Recovered birds do not become carriers of the virus. The resistant nature of the virus to adverse climatic and other influences ensures that the disease is readily perpetuated without the need for carriers.

Rate of spread of the disease varies greatly from flock to flock. In some flocks it is very slow and only a small proportion of the birds become infected. In others dissemination occurs rapidly and practically all the birds become infected in a short time.

Several factors influence rate of spread. Since the virus gains entry to the body through wounds to the skin and mucous membranes, spread is facilitated by conditions which predispose to wounding. These include fighting among birds, the presence of sharp material such as wire, and swallowing of sharp stones and sharp food particles.

Signs

Pox may be seen in birds of any age but is much commoner in adults than in young birds. The level of infection may vary from only a few birds to almost the entire flock. Generally, if affected birds are isolated or culled at an early stage in an outbreak and rigorous hygiene precautions observed, levels of infection can be kept low. However, this depends largely on the virulence of the infecting virus and the degree of resistance of the flock.

Pox occurs in two distinct forms, the skin form and the throat form. Both are commonly seen simultaneously in an outbreak and may even occur together in the same bird.

Skin form

In the skin form, the first sign is the appearance on the wattles and comb of small greyish-white eruptions which become yellow as they rapidly increase in size.

In mild cases, the eruptions may be few in number, but in severe cases large numbers are formed which, as they increase in size, coalesce with neighbouring eruptions to form large, rough wart-like growths which almost completely cover the unfeathered parts of the head. Eruptions may also be found under the wings, around the vent and on the legs and feet.

As the disease progresses the eruptions gradually dry into brown scabs which are surrounded by red areas of inflammation. If the scabs are removed, a raw red surface exuding a watery or purulent fluid will be seen. The scabs normally persist for a few weeks, and in uncomplicated cases they then drop off leaving a smooth scar. Sometimes, however, secondary bacterial infection becomes established which may seriously delay healing of the lesions.

Throat form

In the throat form, the virus invades the cells of the mucous membranes of the mouth and throat, where yellowish-white vesicles form. These soon enlarge, rupture and coalesce to form large areas of dead "cheesy" material, or diphtheritic membranes as such lesions are more properly named. This necrotic material adheres firmly to the underlying tissue and if pulled away leaves a red area of ulceration. Lesions in the mouth may become thickened and dry, eventually, in some cases, preventing closure of the mouth and interfering with eating and swallowing. Again secondary bacterial invasion increases the severity of the condition.

In addition to lesions of pox occurring on the skin and in the mouth, in some birds the facial sinuses are affected resulting in

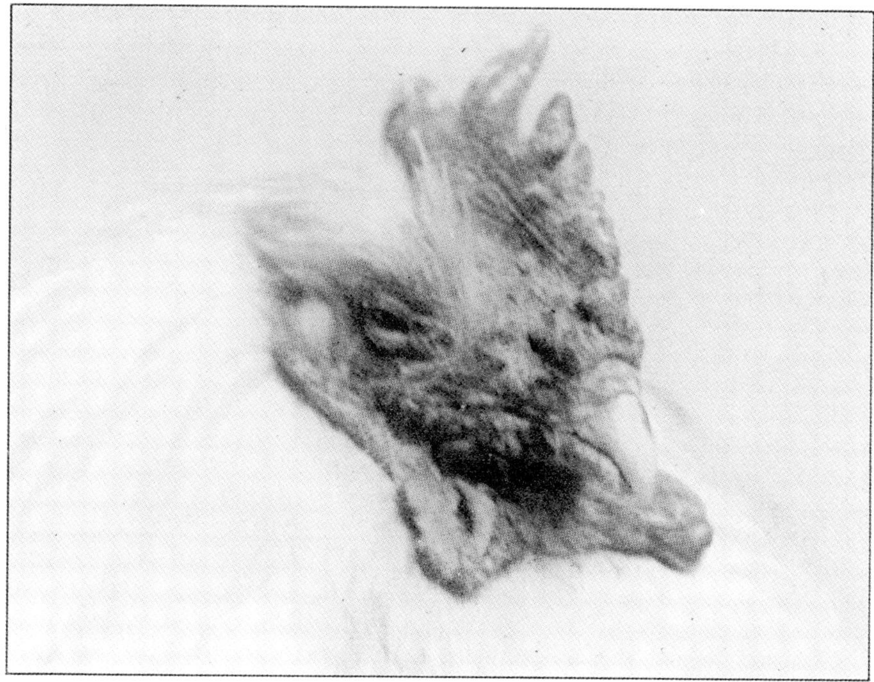

19.1 Comb lesions as a result of fowl pox. Note the whole of the comb and wattles covered with the crusts. The bird has assumed a drowsy attitude tucking the neck well down.

obstruction of the airways and difficulty in breathing. The conjunctivae, or membranes lining the eyes, may also be invaded, resulting in a watery discharge which later becomes purulent, and eventually solid, caseous material accumulates under the eyelids.

Affected birds may show signs of general ill-health, depending on the severity of the condition. In a mild outbreak, particularly if the mouth, throat and sinuses are not affected, no signs of ill-health are seen, but in a severe case there is marked loss of weight and condition, decreased appetite and depression, accompanied by loss of production in laying birds.

Diagnosis

The presence of typical wart-like lesions on the comb and wattles and of yellow caseous accumulations in the mouth and throat is usually sufficient to justify a diagnosis of pox.

Where doubt exists, laboratory tests can be used to confirm the diagnosis. Histological examination of the comb or other affected tissue will show the typical inclusion bodies. Transmission of infec-

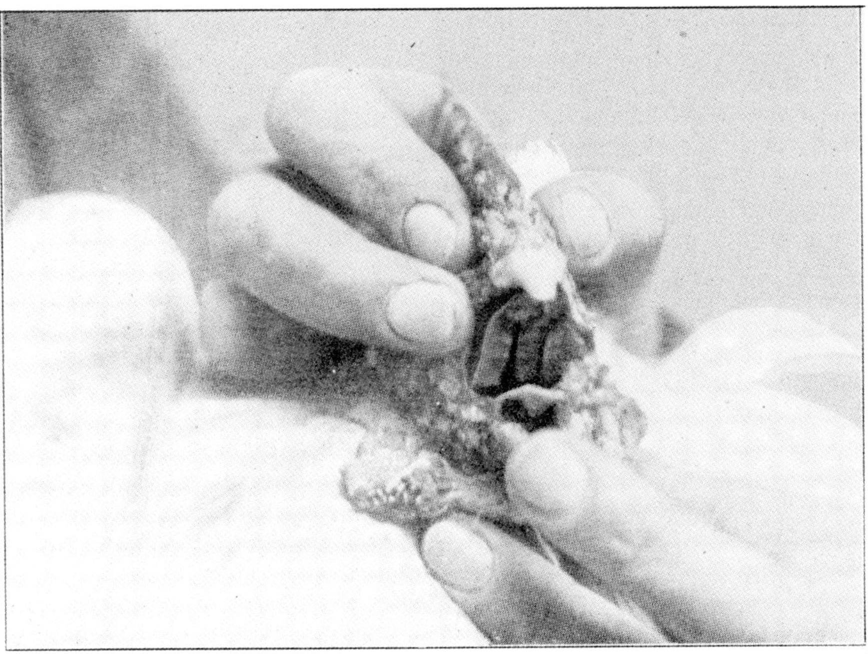

19.2   Fowl Pox: the disease in this case has gradually worked from the comb and wattles, over the beak, into the mouth.

tion to susceptible birds by application of affected tissue to the scarified comb will result in typical disease in these birds, whereas birds protected by previous vaccination and similarly infected will not develop the disease.

Treatment
Drug therapy is of no value in treatment of fowl pox. Antibiotics or other anti-microbials have no effect on the virus. In the event of an outbreak, affected birds should be culled and the remainder of the flock vaccinated. This will give good control of the disease where a slow spreading virus is involved.

In the case of valuable birds, local treatment may be of some value. Caseous material may be removed from affected areas and resulting lesions painted with tincture of iodine or other antiseptic solution or cream. Recovered birds develop a life-long solid immunity to the disease.

As in other infectious diseases, attention to hygiene together with active steps to attempt to prevent spread of infection will have a beneficial effect on the course of an outbreak.

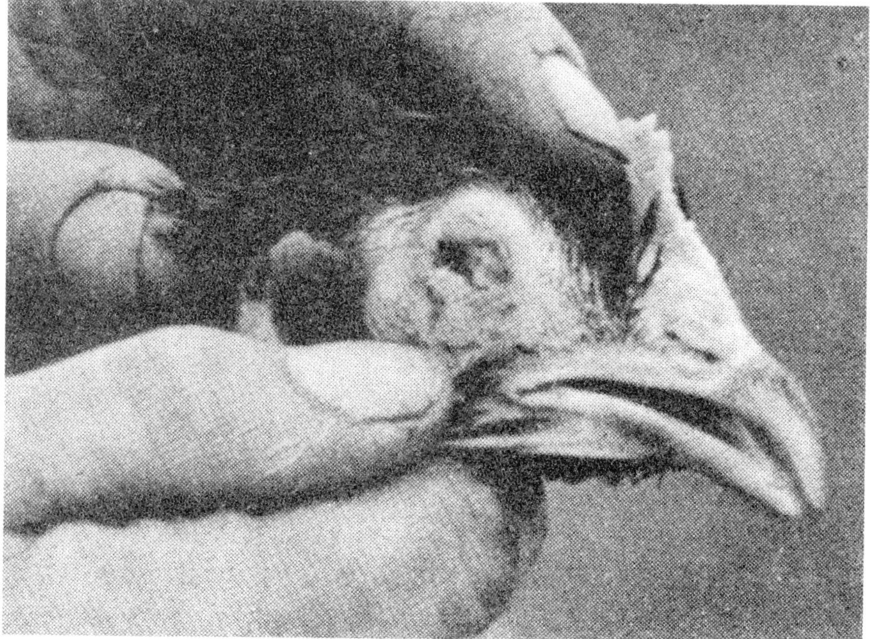

19.3   In some cases of fowl pox the eyes and sinuses of the bird are involved. The eyes become full of pus and bulge outward, and breathing may be affected.

PREVENTION AND CONTROL

As in many other virus diseases, although treatment is of little use, vaccination against the disease results in good immune response and gives satisfactory control.

Modern pox vaccines contain attenuated virus (i.e. the virus used is of reduced virulence for chickens but nevertheless stimulates a strong immune response) and can be given to birds of all ages, including those in lay, but are best administered at six to twelve weeks of age.

There are two principal methods of vaccination; the "stick" method and the "feather-follicle" method. In the **stick method**, several sharp needles mounted together on a base are dipped into the vaccine fluid and then thrust into the skin. The under surface of the web of the wing is the usual site of administration of the vaccine. In the **feather follicle method** a stiff-bristled brush is dipped into the vaccine fluid and then applied to a small region, usually of the thigh, from which the feathers have been removed. The aim is to introduce the virus into the feather follicles. The manufacturer's instructions should always be followed whichever form of vaccination is used.

About a week after vaccination, a sample of birds from the flock are examined to determine whether the vaccination has "taken" as indicated by the presence of a scab at the site of innoculation. If a significant number of birds have failed to develop these lesions, vaccination of these birds should be repeated.

In areas where fowl pox is prevalent, **all birds should be vaccinated** at the appropriate age, but it must be said that at present most of Britain is free of pox and the vast majority of birds are not now vaccinated. In other countries where pox is common all poultry may require to be vaccinated against the disease.

CHAPTER 20

Adenovirus Infections

TYPES

The adenoviruses are common infectious agents of poultry. They can be isolated both from apparently healthy birds and from birds suffering from certain recognisable disease conditions. At present they are being investigated in some detail and certain isolates have been found to be associated with specific diseases.

The original adenovirus isolate was made from human adenoids, hence the name adenovirus. Other isolates were later obtained from mammals and birds. The adenoviruses can, therefore, be divided into two groups depending on whether they are of mammalian or avian origin. Those of avian origin are divided into at least eight serotypes named FAV-1 to FAV-8. Each serotype is further sub-divided into a number of strains, many of which are apparently non-pathogenic but one or two of which can cause disease. Other methods of classifying adenoviruses are being investigated. For example, it is possible to divide strains of various serotypes into two groups depending on nuclear changes and appearances in infected tissue culture cells. Clearly the complex field of avian adenoviruses requires further clarification and indeed a great deal of research effort is going into the study of these common but imperfectly understood infectious agents.

CONDITIONS DUE TO ADENOVIRUSES

The first avian adenovirus isolated was from an epidemic of respiratory disease in quail and was called quail bronchitis virus. This was later shown to be identical to a virus isolated from chicken embryos which was named CELO (chicken embryo lethal orphan). Another adenovirus isolated from chickens was called GAL (gallus adeno-like virus). CELO and GAL are now known to be common infections of chickens but it is generally considered that they have little disease-causing ability and they tend to be disregarded. Some workers however have suggested that they are not entirely innocuous, and it may yet be shown that they have a degree of pathogenicity.

These and other adenovirus isolants have now been made from chickens in many countries and although most are considered non-pathogenic some have been associated with various disease conditions. These include mortality in young chicks, respiratory conditions and drops in egg production. The two diseases most closely associated with adenoviruses however, are **inclusion body hepatitis** and the "newest" disease recorded in Britain which has been called **egg drop syndrome** 1976 or "E.D.S..'76".

INCLUSION BODY HEPATITIS

Nature and Incidence

This disease of broiler chickens has been described in America, Britain and other countries. It is believed to be caused by one or more strains of adenovirus; the **Tipton** strain is usually associated with it and this has been referred to as the **I.B.H. virus**. Other adenovirus strains, however, appear to be involved, and continuing study of this complex problem and further classification of these viruses may eventually shed more light on the precise cause of the disease.

Inclusion body hepatitis is not particularly prevalent in Britain at present but occasional outbreaks occur, typically in broiler birds of about thirty-five to forty-nine days of age. Rarely, pullet flocks may also be affected. Mortality rises quickly to a maximum in about a week, then also falls quickly so that the outbreak is over in a fortnight from the initial deaths. Mortality levels of 5 to 8 per cent are usual but in some cases losses are lower and may be negligible.

Signs

There are no specific signs of the disease before death, although a few birds may be seen to be depressed, standing around with ruffled feathers and closed eyes. Often dead birds are the first indication of the disease in a house.

Cause and related factors

It has been suggested that inclusion body hepatitis is in some way associated with infection by the virus of infectious bursal disease. This disease is known to suppress development of immune mechanisms in young chicks by its effect on the cloacal bursa, the organ mainly responsible for circulating antibody production. The result of this immuno-suppression is that invasion by other infectious agents, including adenoviruses, is facilitated.

A feature of some outbreaks of inclusion body hepatitis is early and marked regression of the cloacal bursa. It may be that this regression is due to early infection by the infectious bursal agent. A similar relationship is believed to exist between infectious bursal disease and gangrenous dermatitis, which is sometimes a complicating factor in outbreaks of inclusion body hepatitis. Research is continuing in an effort to establish the precise relationship between these, and possibly other diseases.

Post Mortem Changes

The main post mortem feature in inclusion body hepatitis is enlargement of the liver, which is yellowish in colour and its surface is mottled with various sized haemorrhages. The kidneys are also enlarged and pale, sometimes with surface haemorrhages and urate deposits in the tubules and ureters. Muscular haemorrhages, particularly in the thigh and breast muscles may also be visible. The cloacal bursa may be reduced in size and firm in consistency. In America, anaemia and pale bone marrow are usually features of the disease but in outbreaks described in Britain these changes were not always present.

Treatment

There is **no specific treatment** for inclusion body hepatitis. Antibiotics have little effect on the course of the disease. Since lateral spread is slow, strict hygienic measures should be helpful. However, the possibility of vertical transmission must be taken into account in control programmes. If, as is suspected, the infectious bursal agent plays a significant part by its immuno-suppressive action on the bursa and lymphatic system, vaccination of parent flocks against this agent could be beneficial by ensuring that high levels of parental antibody are passed to the chick via the egg. This will prevent early infection by the infectious bursal virus and consequent damage to the chicks' immune mechanisms; adequate antibody production against inclusion body hepatitis virus will then occur if the flock should become infected at a later date.

EGG-DROP SYNDROME 1976

One of the commonest problems which face the egg producer and his disease diagnostician is a fall in egg production or, as it is commonly called, an "**egg-drop**". There are many possible causes of this syndrome, such as:
1. Newcastle disease
2. Infectious bronchitis
3. Epidemic tremor
4. Errors in feeding
5. Errors in water supply or lighting
6. Disturbance of birds by livestock
7. Aircraft noise.

In some cases, the cause will be obvious, but in others, even after careful investigation, the cause remains obscure. These production drops have occurred for as long as hens have been kept for the purpose of producing eggs, and will continue to do so. Occasionally, however, a new disease is added to the list of those responsible for production drops. The most recent of these made its appearance in the U.K. and Ireland in 1976, and since then has caused a good deal of trouble in the industry and has received considerable publicity.

Nature and Incidence

The disease is believed to be caused by an adenovirus (although some say that this is not yet entirely proven), the isolates recovered in Ireland and England being called "**127**" and "**BC 14**" respectively. These are now known to be identical viruses and the disease itself has been called **Egg-drop Syndrome 1976** (or "E.D.S.76"). The virus, although classed as an adenovirus differs from other fowl adenoviruses in certain respects, chiefly in its ability to agglutinate fowl red blood corpuscles. The possession of this property means that a haemagglutination inhibition test is available for laboratory diagnosis of the disease.

A condition similar to E.D.S.76 was apparently present in the Netherlands for some time previously, but within the British Isles it first made its appearance in Ireland in the summer of 1976 and occurred shortly afterwards in England. The disease affected mainly broiler parent stock of one large breeding organisation and was characterised by production drops of as much as 30 to 50 per cent occurring invariably close to the time of peak production, mainly between the ages of twenty-eight to thirty-two weeks. In other cases, instead of drops in production, flocks simply failed to achieve expected production peaks. This syndrome differed from previously known causes of loss of production in that these might occur at any time after birds are in lay, rather than in association with peak production in every case.

Signs

Affected flocks apparently show little evidence of any upset in general health apart from a transient diarrhoea (which has never been proven to be part of the syndrome). There is, however, a pronounced effect on shell quality of eggs laid during an outbreak. This may range from paleness with loss of bloom to soft shelled or shell-less eggs. Another feature of this disease which distinguishes it from other causes of production drops is that these shell changes are frequently noted *before* the loss of production occurs. In the Netherlands, internal egg quality has also been affected; cloudy and watery thin albumen have been recorded. This has not been a feature of cases in the U.K.. Egg quality effects are short-lived, occurring only for a brief period in the early stages of the disease. Egg production however may not return to normal for two months or more.

Diagnosis

Diagnosis of the disease is mainly an exercise in differentiating it from other causes of loss of production. The features already mentioned, supported by laboratory demonstration of antibodies in blood samples taken from the suspect flock are good evidence on which to base a diagnosis.

Origin

The precise origin of the virus is still uncertain but its sudden appearance almost simultaneously in birds of one breed in Ireland and England, and other circumstantial evidence, has given rise to the suggestion that it was a contaminant of a live virus vaccine. This has not been proved, but it underlines the importance of purity of live vaccines and the ever-present possibility that a previously unknown agent could be introduced by this means to a susceptible population.

Spread

Spread of the virus is believed to occur from dam to offspring by vertical transmission through the egg. When the condition first appeared it was noted that lateral spread, if it occurred at all, was slow if birds were separated by a wire partition. This is probably still true, but there is evidence that lateral spread is now becoming more rapid. Certainly, spread from bird to bird within a pen occurs rapidly; it is believed that the virus is passed with the droppings and that this is a more significant means of spread than the air-borne route.

In some flocks, it can be shown by blood testing that antibodies are present in the blood before the flock comes into production. In others, antibodies do not become demonstrable until after egg laying commences. It is believed that the virus, although present in these latter flocks, remains in a latent or dormant state until activated by the stress of production. A number of measures based on the epidemiology of the disease can be undertaken in an effort to limit spread. Since lateral spread is slow, good hygiene and efficient disease control measures should be effective. In particular, since faecal spread is believed to be important in dissemination of the virus, it is important that attendants should change footwear and protective clothing before moving from one flock or house to another on a site. Care should be taken that the virus is not spread by such operations as blood testing or vaccinating. It is believed that parent birds of forty weeks and over no longer transmit virus through the egg, so that hatching of eggs only from flocks over this age should prevent vertical transmission. However, where hatching of eggs from infected parent flocks is essential, these should be hatched separately from eggs derived from non-infected parent.

Prevention

Probably the best way for a poultry farmer to avoid E.D.S. infection is to take stock only from known uninfected parents which in turn have been derived from uninfected grandparents and to practise efficient disease control methods. In this way both vertical and lateral transmission is avoided. However, these ideal measures may not always be practicable. In Ireland, the disease has apparently been eradicated by hatching only from birds of over forty weeks, serological testing and exercising best possible disease control measures. There the disease occurred mainly in broiler parents; in England it now occurs also in commercial layers and their parents. It remains to be seen whether attempts to control the disease will be as successful in England, where a vaccine has been developed and is now in use as an additional control measure. The vaccine is given by injection between fourteen and eighteen weeks of age and has been successful in preventing production drops. It does not, however, prevent infected birds excreting virus and, because it may mask infection, it has been suggested that its use in parent flocks should be avoided. There is at present some evidence that infection in commercial laying birds is becoming more widespread and it appears that unless the infection can be rapidly controlled and eliminated by whatever means, the poultry industry will have to accept and learn to live with this new pathogen.

Up until recently there was no evidence that the disease occurs in areas of the world other than the British Isles and the Netherlands. Care should be taken to ensure that it is not introduced to other areas by export of birds hatched from infected flocks. (However, since this was written, serological evidence of the infection has come to light in other countries including the U.S.A. and Nigeria.)

CHAPTER 21

Marek's Disease

NATURE AND TYPE

Marek's disease is a virus induced neoplastic or cancerous disease of the domestic chicken. Formerly known as **fowl paralysis** it was included along with several other apparently related diseases in the so-called **Avian Leucosis Complex**. Much research effort has gone into the study of this disease complex for many years and as the nature and cause of the various diseases have been elucidated the term Avian Leucosis Complex has now become obsolete.

The use of the term Avian Leucosis Complex resulted from the fact that a number of diseases of the fowl showed similar pathological changes which made diagnosis of individual diseases, their separation from other diseases and investigation of their causes matters of great difficulty. The original work on the complex was performed by Dr. J. Marek in Hungary in the early years of this century. He used the term **poly-neuritis** to describe a lameness in chickens. Additional work was carried on by a great many eminent scientists in many countries. Many other terms for diseases within the complex were used and much confusion resulted. It was not until the nineteen-sixties that the diseases and their causes were finally separated and it was shown that the two most important diseases within the Avian Leucosis Complex are Marek's disease and **lymphoid leucosis**. It was demonstrated that the diseases are caused by distinct and separate viruses and that lymphoid leucosis is egg-transmitted while Marek's disease is not. Lymphoid leucosis and the other leucoses are considered in the next chapter.

Incidence

Marek's disease is world-wide in distribution and has been the cause of severe economic loss to the poultry industries of many countries. The production of a vaccine against the disease was one of the most outstanding achievements in the control of poultry diseases. The use of this vaccine which became available in the early nineteen–seventies has greatly reduced the incidence of the disease in Britain and many other countries. There has not been a corresponding reduction in the amount of Marek's disease virus in the environment and it is apparent that vaccination will continue to be necessary for many years to come if the disease is to be kept under control.

Cause

Marek's disease is caused by a herpes virus which, when it infects the chicken, stimulates enormous multiplication of certain cells which closely resemble the lymphocytes of the white blood cell series. These cells accumulate in various organs and nerve trunks in the bird's body giving rise to enlargement of affected organs and thickening of nerves.

Source of Outbreaks

Marek's disease virus is extremely prevalent in poultry populations on a world wide basis. In contrast to the virus of lymphoid leucosis it is not vertically transmitted through the egg so that at hatching chicks are free of infection. They are most susceptible within the first few weeks of life however, and contact with the virus during this stage will result in infection. The virus has been shown to be present in high concentration in feather follicle epithelium of infected birds, and feather dust or "dander" is the most important means by which the virus is transmitted from infected to non-infected birds and by which the environment becomes contaminated. The virus requires the protection provided by these cells to survive in the environment and in this protected state it can survive for periods up to one year. The actual method of spread of the disease is believed to be by **inhalation of this feather dust containing the virus**, infection gaining entry to the blood stream via the respiratory tract. Infection then generally persists for the life of the bird with continuous shedding of the virus into the environment via the feather dust. **The importance of contamination of the environment in the transfer of infection to young chicks cannot be overemphasised.**

COURSE AND NATURE OF MAREK'S DISEASE

Infection with Marek's disease virus takes place early in the bird's life, usually in the first few days and almost certainly within the first eight weeks. However, infection is followed by a long incubation period so that clinical signs are not seen until about six weeks of age at the earliest and more commonly not until twelve weeks or later.

Two Types

Two more or less distinct clinical types of Marek's disease occur. The first, known as **neural of classical** Marek's disease follows infiltration of proliferating lymphocytes into nerve trunks and results in paralysis of wings, legs, neck etc., depending on which nerves are affected. The second type, known as **visceral or acute** Marek's disease is due to accumulation of lymphocytes in various internal organs resulting in development of lymphomatous tumours in these organs. It must be emphasised that while in many outbreaks of the disease one or other type may predominate there is no clear-cut division between the two. Some nerve involvement may occur in outbreaks of the acute form and tumours are often seen in a few birds in outbreaks of the classical form.

The duration of the disease and the mortality in an affected flock are variable. In some cases only a few birds are lost over a period of a week or two while in others birds continue to die for many weeks or months. Losses are generally higher in outbreaks of the acute form. Several factors are known to influence the number of birds affected and the losses in an outbreak. These include the genetic susceptibility to the disease of the birds in the flock, their age and sex and whether or not they were vaccinated against the disease. Also of great importance is the strain and virulence of the particular virus causing an outbreak.

Susceptibility

The degree of susceptibility depends on the breed and strain of bird involved. Birds which are genetically resistant have the ability to resist development of the disease after infection, not to resist infection itself. The sex of the chicken is important in that females are more susceptible than males, the ovary being affected by tumours much more frequently than the testes.

Chickens are more susceptible to Marek's disease in early life and resistance increases with age. For this reason **vaccination must be performed as early as possible** in order to protect the chick at the most vulnerable stage in its life.

The strain of infecting virus may determine whether or not Marek's disease develops in a flock. Not all naturally-occurring strains will induce disease, and indeed some non-pathogenic strains may induce resistance in infected birds to other more virulent strains, without themselves causing any ill effects. Infection of susceptible birds by virulent strains, on the other hand may give rise to either the classical form or the acute form of the disease.

In addition to these specific factors, it should be mentioned that any form of stress applied to a flock may convert a dormant Marek's disease infection to an active infection, probably by reducing the birds' resistance to the disease. It is often noted that outbreaks occur in pullet flocks shortly after they come into egg production. In these cases the stress of production itself may be the precipitating factor or it may be that moving of birds to laying quarters, change of food, etc., at this time are important influences.

Signs

The signs shown by an individual bird depend on which form of disease is present, classical or acute. In many outbreaks both types are present so that signs are variable. When the classical (neural) form predominates, the main signs are paralysis of wings, legs or occasionally other areas of the body depending on which nerves are affected. Thus birds may be seen with dropped wings, off their legs or they may have twisted necks. If the nerves to the bowel are affected diarrhoea may be present. Occasionally respiratory signs are present when the intercostal nerves are involved. When birds are seen off their legs a characteristic attitude is often adopted of one leg stretched forward and the other backwards. When two or three birds are seen in this posture it is almost diagnostic of Marek's disease.

In the acute form of the disease there may be no specific signs but some birds can usually be seen to be depressed, poorly grown and in poor condition. Others may die with no preceding signs. In both forms of the disease, but particularly in the acute type, if death is delayed by more than a few days, loss of weight often occurs, sometimes to the point of emaciation.

Mortality is usually higher in the acute form of the disease. It may be 10 to 30 per cent or even higher. In the classical type, mortality rarely exceeds 10 per cent.

Post Mortem Findings

The post mortem findings in birds dead of Marek's disease also

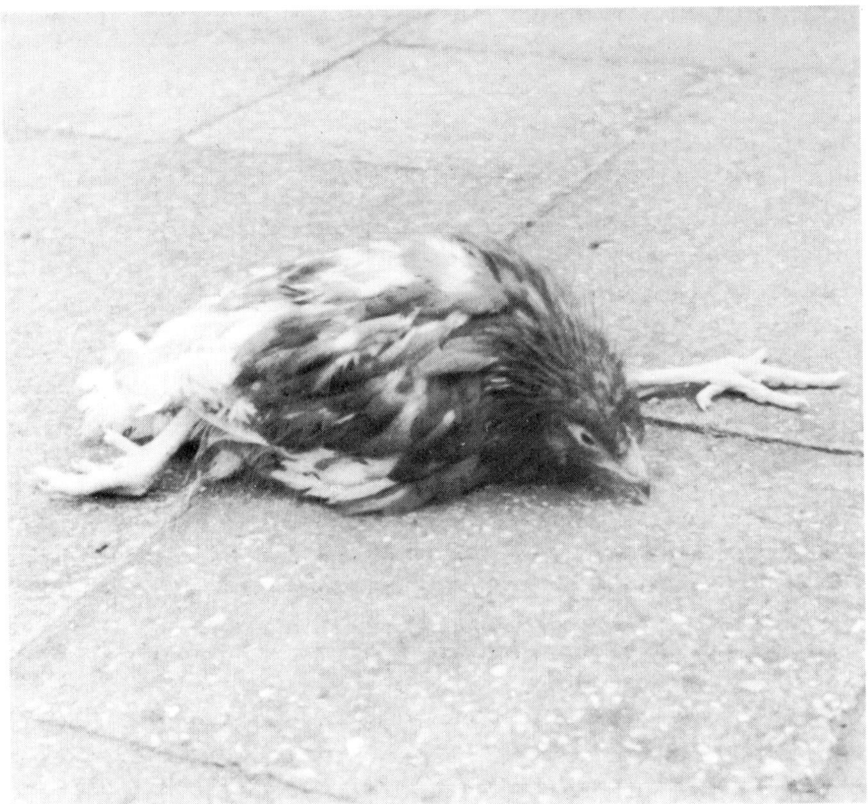

21.1 Typical attitude in neural Marek's disease. One leg stretched forward, the other back.

depend on the type of disease. In the classical form, the main change is enlargement and thickening of various nerve plexuses and trunks. Those most commonly affected are the brachial plexus which controls the wings and the sciatic plexus and nerves which control the legs. Also frequently involved are the vagus nerve, the coeliac plexus and the splanchnic nerves.

Affected nerves may be three times normal thickness or more; they lose their normal glistening appearance and become grey or yellowish in colour. Changes in nerves are often unilateral so that the nerves on both sides of the body should always be examined.

In the acute form of the disease, the main finding is lymphoid tumour formation in various organs throughout the bird's body. Tumours are most commonly found in the ovary, liver, spleen, heart, lungs and proventriculus. Sometimes the kidneys are involved and tumours may also occur in the skin and in the muscles.

Affected organs are enlarged sometimes to several times their normal size, assume a uniform grey colour and become firm in consistency. In the liver there may be multiple nodular growths or the organs may be diffusely involved and uniformly enlarged. Nodular growths are often present in the heart. When the proventriculus is involved it is obviously enlarged and the internal surface may be red and ulcerated. Skin growths occur as small white nodules associated with feather follicles, and muscle tumours are small nodules or large firm masses.

Birds which have died of Marek's disease are often in extremely poor condition with prominent breast bone and loss of muscle volume. If birds were unable to reach water before death, dehydration of the carcase may be noticeable.

Diagnosis

Diagnosis of Marek's disease in most cases presents little difficulty. The ante mortem signs and post mortem changes are characteristic and should give rise to immediate suspicion of the disease. There is however one major difficulty in diagnosis, namely that the lesions of lymphoid leucosis are in many cases identical to, or so closely similar to those of Marek's disease that it is impossible to differentiate the diseases on clinical signs and post mortem examination. There may on occasion be good reason for making such a diagnosis, for example, in cases of Marek's disease vaccine breakdown, (i.e. occurrence of Marek's disease in birds which were previously vaccinated against the disease) it is obviously important to ensure that the disease being investigated is in fact Marek's and not leucosis.

There are, however, a number of distinguishing features between the two conditions which should be considered when making a diagnosis. The most important of these are the presence or absence of nerve involvement, the age at which the disease occurs, the distribution of lesions, the involvement of the bursa of Fabricius and the type of cell visible on histological examination of affected tissues

Nerve involvement occurs only in Marek's disease, and while lymphoid leucosis is almost never seen at less than sixteen weeks of age, Marek's disease may be seen from about six weeks onwards. In Marek's disease lesions may be seen in many organs and tissues while in leucosis lesions are confined mainly, although not exclusively, to the liver and spleen. The bursa may be involved in both diseases but in leucosis the tumours tend to be nodular while in Marek's disease the bursa is diffusely enlarged. In Marek's disease the skin, muscle tissue and proventriculus may show tumour formation while in leucosis these sites are rarely if ever involved.

It will be seen that in most cases a diagnosis can be made from a consideration of these features. Thus if disease is present in birds of less than sixteen weeks of age, if nerve lesions occur or if tumours are present in skin, muscle or proventriculus the condition is almost certainly Marek's disease. It is in cases where the disease is first seen in birds of over sixteen weeks and in which no nerve involvement or distinctive tumours are present that difficulties arise. In these cases histological examination of affected tissues is necessary to arrive at a precise diagnosis. The diseases can be differentiated by the type of cell predominating in histological preparations, but a good deal of experience is required on the part of the pathologist if an accurate diagnosis is to be made by this means.

PREVENTION AND CONTROL

No treatment is of any value in birds affected by Marek's disease; such **birds should be culled**. The main method of prevention is the use of live virus vaccines now available against the disease. Because infection is acquired by chicks in early life, vaccination must be performed as soon as possible after hatching and in practice the vaccine is normally administered at one day old, before chicks leave the hatchery. Vaccination has proved highly effective and has dramatically reduced losses from the disease, but to be fully successful, it should be supplemented by correct management procedures. Thorough cleaning and disinfection of the poultry house before chicks are introduced is necessary, and an "all-in, all-out" system should be adopted where possible. It is on multi-age sites where chicks are reared in close proximity to older birds that vaccination failures and outbtreaks of the disease are most likely to occur. Chicks should certainly be reared separately from older birds for the first few weeks of life while they are most susceptible to infection by the virus. Careful attention to hygiene and management will help to ensure that chicks do not meet the highly infectious disease agent before the vaccine has had time to confer a useful degree of immunity.

At one time breeding organisations engaged in a programme of selection for genetic resistance to the disease but since the introduction of vaccination this method of attempted control has been dropped.

As stated, Marek's disease vaccine is normally administered in the hatchery. The vaccine is injected intra-muscularly or subcutaneously, the dose being 0.2 ml.. The manufacturer's instructions should be carefully followed when preparing the vaccine for use. Vaccines available in Britain contain a herpes virus of turkey origin which is non-pathogenic to turkeys and chickens but which confers immunity to Marek's disease when administered to chickens. **Two types of vaccine** are available, a "**cell-associated**" vaccine which must be stored in liquid nitrogen, and a freeze-dried "**cell-free**" vaccine which is stored in the refrigerator at 2° to 6°C. Most companies now produce the freeze-dried vaccine. In some other countries, vaccines containing modified Marek's disease virus are used.

Vaccine failures

Although vaccination against Marek's disease has dramatically reduced the incidence of disease, naturally occurring virus is still widespread and any unvaccinated flock is almost equally at risk now as in pre-vaccination days. In addition, vaccine failures or "breaks" in vaccinated flocks occasionally occur, to the consternation of the flock owner who is rather inclined to take for granted the efficacy of the vaccine and may find difficulty in accepting even a low incidence of the disease in a vaccinated flock.

The reasons for vaccine breaks have been diligently sought. Although a number of possibilities exist there is no doubt that one of the most important factors is severe disease challenge before vaccinal immunity has had time to develop. This is likely where a high concentration of Marek's disease virus exists on a poultry farm due to the operation of a continuous production system, where houses are inadequately disinfected before chicks are placed and where other hygiene measures are lacking.

The possibility that maternal antibodies against turkey herpes virus (i.e. vaccine virus), transferred from breeder birds to chicks via the yolk, may interfere with vaccinal immunity has been considered. This however is now believed to be a relatively unimportant cause of vaccine failure.

Other possible causes of vaccine breaks relate to handling, storage and administration of vaccine. The vaccine must be stored as recommended by the manufacturers and made up in the diluent supplied. After dilution it must be used within six hours. The number of chicks which can be vaccinated in a given time depends on the skill of the vaccinator, but about one thousand per hour appears to be a safe maximum where a syringe is used. Recently, vaccination machines have been used which can probably double this rate of administration. If vaccinating personnel try to increase beyond reasonable limits the number of chicks vaccinated in a fixed time, there is a definite possibility of mistakes occurring. Boxes of chicks or individuals may be missed, vaccine may not be properly administered and so on. A well-trained and supervised team will avoid these errors.

It is a measure of the success of Marek's disease vaccination that farmers now consider unacceptable losses from the disease which, in pre-vaccination days, would have been regarded as relatively light and unavoidable. Although in a few individual cases mortality can still be high, one of the greatest scourges of the poultry industry has been reduced, on a national scale, to a disease of minor importance. It must be repeated however that virulent virus is still present in the chicken population and no relaxation of the present vaccination policy can be foreseen at present.

The remarks regarding vaccination apply particularly to pullets, but there is some evidence that vaccination of broilers will result in better performance even though it is unlikely that clinical disease will occur in unvaccinated broilers due to the early age at which they are killed. Those engaged in producing pure breeds for commercial purposes or as a hobby should note that their birds, some of which may be of considerable individual value, are at risk if they fail to provide the protection afforded by Mareks disease vaccination.

Following an outbreak of the disease thorough disinfection of the poultry house is necessary. Adoption of an "all-in, all-out" system along with adequate hygiene measures should result in satisfactory control of the disease, although the highly infectious nature of the virus and its prevalence in poultry populations means that infection of succeeding chick flocks is an ever present hazard.

CHAPTER 22

Lymphoid Leucosis and other Leucoses

NATURE AND INCIDENCE

Lymphoid leucosis is another virus-induced lymphoid neoplastic condition within the Avian Leucosis Complex. The causative virus, however, belongs to the leucosis sarcoma group and is totally distinct from that of Marek's disease. Unlike Marek's disease, the virus of lymphoid leucosis is passed through the egg and this is the main method of transmission of the disease. Although the virus is widespread in poultry populations, outbreaks of the disease are sporadic and mortality is usually much less than in the case of Marek's disease. Nevertheless high mortality can occur in individual flocks on occasion. Lymphoid leucosis is the only disease within the leucosis complex other than Marek's disease which is of economic significance. It is the main subject of this chapter; the other leucoses are considered briefly at the end.

Source of Outbreaks

As mentioned, the virus of lymphoid leucosis is egg transmitted; infected parent birds transmit the virus to their progeny, and these infected birds shed the virus in their saliva and droppings, thus transmitting infection to their pen mates and other birds in the locality. However, the virus does not survive long outside the chicken's body so that lateral transmission is probably of minor importance. Practically all commercial flocks become infected by lymphoid leucosis virus but only a small number of infected birds develop the disease. Resistance to infection increases with age.

COURSE OF THE DISEASE

Although lymphoid leucosis is egg transmitted so that chicks are infected at hatching, clinical disease and mortality rarely occur at less than sixteen weeks of age. The virus infects many organs of the bird's body but the organ in which neoplastic transformation occurs is the cloacal bursa. The virus induces cancerous change in the bursa at perhaps four weeks of age in chicks which were infected by vertical transmission, and as in Marek's disease the neoplastic cells are white blood cells of the lymphocyte series, although the predominant cell type or lymphoblast is a less mature form than in Marek's disease. These transformed cells remain in a dormant state until the bird is sixteen weeks or older when they are released from the bursa and invade other organs, especially the liver and spleen, resulting in massive enlargement of these organs and eventual death. Not all infected birds develop lesions or die of the disease, however; some become healthy carriers and shedders of the virus, and these birds can contaminate the environment or transmit the disease to their offspring via the egg.

Susceptibility
Whether or not a bird develops lymphoid leucosis after infection depends on several factors. Some birds have a genetic resistance to the disease, others are fully susceptible. Chicks infected via the egg are more likely to succumb to the disease than those infected by contact. Younger chicks are more susceptible than older birds although antibodies derived from the parent bird give the chick some protection for the first week or two of life. Finally, the dose of virus is important; as might be expected, the higher the dose of virus acquired by a chick, whatever the means of infection, the more likely the chick is to develop the disease.

Signs
There are no specific signs of the disease. Birds may be found dead while still in good condition. Others become weak, with loss of appetite, pale comb and wattles and general emaciation. Handling individual birds may reveal an enlarged liver. There are **no signs referable to nerve involvement** as occur in Marek's disease.

Signs and mortality in lymphoid leucosis invariably occur after sixteen weeks of age and often after birds come into lay; a low, persistent level of mortality usually continues until the flock is past peak production.

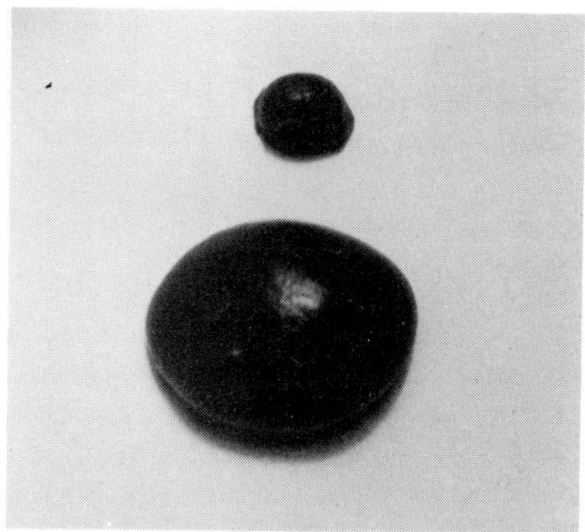

22.1 Grossly enlarged spleen from case of lymphoid leucosis compared with normal spleen.

Post Mortem Findings

The main post mortem changes are found in internal organs, particularly the liver and spleen. These organs are enlarged sometimes up to several times their normal size. The liver is pale in colour. Usually the whole organ is uniformly and diffusely enlarged but a nodular type of involvement is common in which large or small nodular tumours are scattered throughout the liver substance. Diffuse or nodular involvement of the spleen may occur. Other organs including ovary, kidneys and lungs may also be affected although less regularly than in Marek's disease. In lymphoid leucosis a tumour is almost invariably present in the cloacal bursa. Sometimes this can be seen on gross post mortem but often microscopic examination is required to reveal it.

Diagnosis

The clinical signs, mortality level, age of bird affected and post mortem changes should enable the clinician to suspect lymphoid leucosis. The main diagnostic difficulty is differentiation between this disease and certain cases of Marek's disease, particularly those in which losses begin after sixteen weeks and in which no nervous signs or lesions are present. Definitive diagnosis of such cases can be difficult and histological examination of affected tissues may be necessary to differentiate between the two diseases. A brief account of the main distinguishing features is given in the chapter on Marek's disease.

It is unlikely that lymphoid leucosis lesions would be confused with those of other conditions although they may bear some resemblance to the lesions of certain cases of tuberculosis. Staining of smears in the laboratory for the presence of the acid-fast organisms of tuberculosis will quickly differentiate these diseases.

Although blood tests for lymphoid leucosis exist, they are of little value for diagnosis of the disease because of the high proportion of birds which are infected but which show no signs of disease; blood tests are likely to be positive whether birds tested are suffering from the disease or not.

Treatment and Control

There is **no useful treatment** for lymphoid leucosis; affected **birds should be culled** and their carcases disposed of.

There is **no vaccine** available for protection against the disease. It should be clearly understood that, although lymphoid leucosis and Marek's disease are clinically similar conditions, the two are separate and distinct diseases, and **Marek's disease vaccines does not protect against lymphoid leucosis.** The only practical methods of prevention involve maintaining high standards of hygiene in order to reduce the risk of lateral infection from the environment. Rearing of chicks away from older birds is advisable although, because the disease is egg transmitted, isolation rearing will not prevent infection unless chicks are acquired from a disease-free source. This is not generally possible under commercial conditions at the present time. However, investigations are taking place into methods of producing disease-free flocks. Recent advances in detection of infected birds suggest that eradication of disease from breeding flocks may eventually become a practical proposition. Egg transmission would thereby be prevented and it would be a relatively easy matter to prevent infection of chicks from lateral sources in view of the short survival time of the virus outside the body.

Recently, a drug known as **mibolerone** added to the food of infected chicks, has been shown to reduce the incidence of lymphoid leucosis by causing regression of the cloacal bursa, the organ in which the primary lesion orginates. Investigations into its use under practical conditions are taking place.

OTHER LEUCOSES

In addition to lymphoid leucosis, a number of other viral induced leucotic conditions of chickens exist, the principal difference being that in these conditions **cells of the blood other than the lymphocytes** are involved. In **erythroleucosis,** the cells affected are immature red cells or erythroblasts while in **myeloid leucosis,** immature or mature cells of the granular white cell series are involved. Myeloid leucosis is further divided into **myelobastosis** and **myelocytomatosis** depending on whether immature or mature granulocytes are affected. In addition, there is another condition known as **osteopetrosis** in which the bones of the legs become greatly thickened. These conditions are extremely rare in comparison with lymphoid leucosis and are of little economic significance. It should be recalled that all these conditions, including Mareks disease were grouped together in the avian leucosis complex before their separate viral causes were properly understood, and indeed the term avian leucosis complex is still sometimes used to refer to this group of diseases.

Indications and post mortem features

The main clinical and post mortem features of erythroleucosis are similar to those of lymphoid leucosis, the principle difference being a distinct cherry red colour of the liver, spleen and bone marrow which is due to accumulation of large numbers of immature red cells within the blood vessels of these organs. This colour contrasts with the pale, creamy-white colour of the tumours of Marek's disease and the other leucoses.

In myeloblastosis the liver and spleen are again greatly enlarged, the liver having a Morocco-leather appearance and a granular consistency. Meylocytomatosis is also characterised by enlarged liver and spleen but the tumours these organs contain are discrete and nodular. In addition, tumours frequently occur in the flat bones of the skull, ribs and breast-bone in this condition.

There is no treatment for any of these diseases. They are so rare that preventive measures are scarcely warranted, although the principles mentioned under lymphoid leucosis would apply.

LEUCOSIS IN TURKEYS

It has been known for a good many years that turkeys are occasionally affected by a condition which is closely similar to leucosis of the chicken. It appears that at least two distinct conditions occur in turkeys, both viral induced, one being referred to as **lymphoproliferative disease** and the other as **reticuloendotheliosis**. These conditions occur sporadically but can be

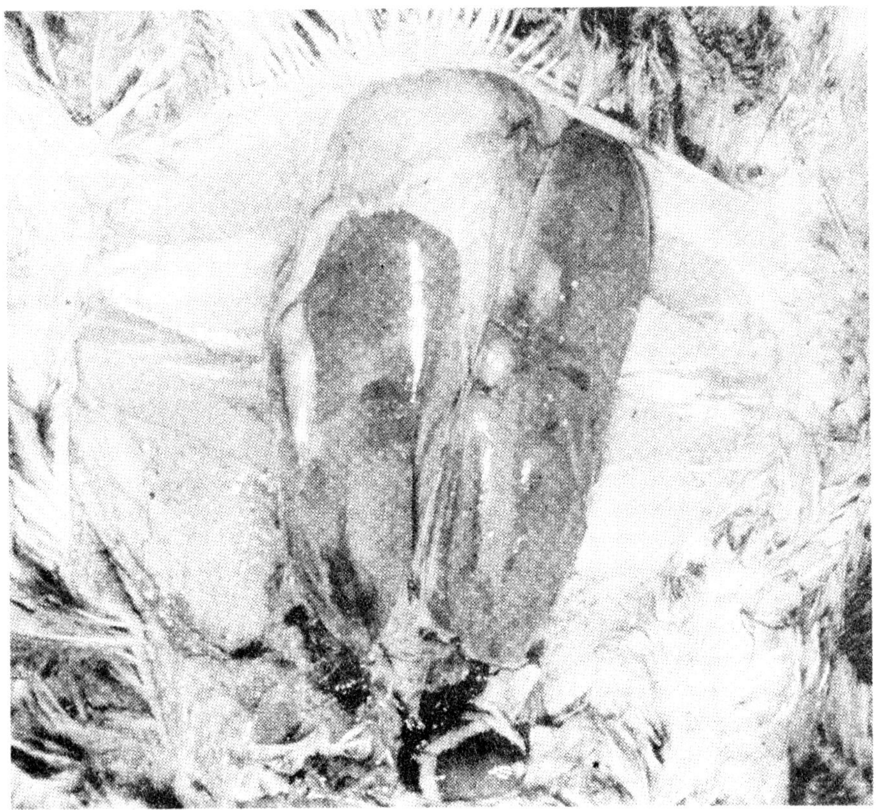

22.2 Leucosis of the liver. The organ is grossly enlarged and almost fills the abdomen.

responsible for significant mortality in affected flocks. Birds over ten weeks of age are usually affected.

The post mortem picture is similar to lymphoid leucosis in the chicken with enlarged spleen and liver containing multiple lymphoid tumours. Tumours may also occur in other organs and sometimes nerve trunks are affected as in Marek's disease.

Further work is required to elucidate the precise nature of these leucosis-like diseases in turkeys.

CHAPTER 23

Other Viral Diseases

This chapter deals with four viral diseases which are of significance to the poultry keeper. They are:

1. **Duck virus hepatitis**
2. **Duck virus enteritis**
3. **Avian Influenza and Fowl Plague**
4. **Haemorrhagic Enteritis of Turkeys**

Each is described in detail in the following sections.

DUCK VIRUS HEPATITIS

Nature and Incidence

This is an acute, highly fatal disease of ducklings which was first described in Long Island U.S.A. in 1950 and has since occurred in many countries of the world including Britain. Chickens, turkeys and other birds are resistant to the disease. It is restricted to young ducklings particularly those under three weeks of age. Adult ducks on infected premises have never shown any signs of ill-health, while their egg production, fertility and hatchability have remained unimpaired.

Signs

Duck virus hepatitis is characterised by its sudden onset, rapid spread among susceptible ducklings and high mortality. Introduction of the disease to a flock may be by contaminated food, water or equipment; wild birds, including wild ducks may on occasion act as carriers of the virus. Bird-to-bird spread then occurs by faecal contamination of food, litter, etc. Recovered ducklings do not appear to become carriers of the disease, virus being excreted only up to about fifteen days after the onset of signs. However, litter from infected pens has been found to be infective ten weeks after ducklings suffering from virus hepatitis were removed.

The course of the disease in fully susceptible ducklings is extremely rapid; birds die within perhaps an hour or two of first showing signs. Affected birds become dull and listless, stand with eyes closed, very soon go over on their sides and make spasmodic paddling movements with their legs; death follows rapidly. A characteristic sign in this disease is that shortly before death, birds arch their necks so that the head is drawn backwards to a position on the back almost between the wings. This sign is correctly referred to as **opisthotonus** and its appearance in a highly acute and fatal disease of ducklings should give rise to immediate suspicion of virus hepatitis.

Post mortem changes and diagnosis

Post mortem changes are found mainly in the liver, which is enlarged with haemorrhages scattered over its surface, or in some cases a generalised reddish mottling of the liver surface will be seen. The spleen and kidneys are also enlarged in many cases.

Diagnosis of the disease can usually be made from the characteristic signs and post mortem changes. Confirmation of diagnosis in the laboratory depends on innoculation of material from affected ducklings into embryonating hens' eggs, with deaths and certain changes in the embryos visible after several more days incubation.

Treatment

There is **no useful treatment** for affected birds. Spread is generally so rapid that hygiene or other control methods are ineffective. In America, **immune serum** treatment is used. A bank of this serum, collected from birds which have suffered from or been vaccinated against the disease, is kept in readiness for use in outbreaks; it contains antibodies against the disease and injection gives immediate protection. It must be used as early as possible in the course of an outbreak to save the maximum number of birds. This is one of the few instances of use of an antiserum, as distinct from a vaccine, in the field of avian medicine. It has the advantage of giving immediate protection, whereas a vaccine requires a variable amount of time for protection to build up. In dealing with a highly acute disease such as duck virus hepatitis, even if vaccination is performed in the earliest possible stage of an outbreak, many birds may die before the vaccine stimulates protection, simply because of the associated time lag.

Prevention

Vaccination is, however, also used to protect ducklings against virus hepatitis. It may be administered to breeding stock which develop antibodies against the disease and pass these to the offspring via the egg. These maternally immune ducklings may, in addition, be vaccinated at ten days of age, this regime giving protection for the critical three week period. In the case of ducklings hatched from non-immune parents, vaccination should be done when day old to give earliest possible protection.

The method of vaccination is by puncture of the foot-web by a needle dipped in a suspension of attenuated virus. Usually a single vaccination gives sufficient protection.

DUCK VIRUS ENTERITIS

Nature and Incidence

This is another important virus disease of ducks which has been reported from many countries, particularly the Netherlands and the Long Island duck producing area of the U.S.A.. The disease has occurred in Britain, but only in a small number of pond birds. Major commercial enterprises were not affected.

Duck virus enteritis, known also as **Duck Plague,** is an acute, highly contagious disease of ducks, geese and swans. Other types of poultry are resistant. The disease may affect any age of birds (in contrast to duck virus hepatitis), spreads by direct contact or by indirect transfer of virus and is apparently more prevalent in ducks which have access to water. It is believed that infected pond water is one of the main means of transmission of the disease.

Signs

Signs of duck virus enteritis include loss of appetite, thirst, depression, nasal discharge, sticky discharge from the eyes with, in some cases, closed eyelids, diarrhoea and nervous signs of imbalance and inability to stand. A blue colour of the beak may be seen and in some cases the droppings contain blood which stains the vent feathers.

In adult birds the first indication of the disease may be sudden mortality accompanied by a sharp drop in egg production.

Post Mortem Changes

Post mortem changes in duck virus enteritis involve many organs and are rather characteristic. The disease affects the blood vascular system, with multiple haemorrhages in many organs being the main lesion. Haemorrhages of varying size may be found on the heart, liver, kidneys and lungs and in the wall of the intestine. In laying birds, the ovaries may be haemorrhagic and discoloured. Haemorrhagic rings in the lymphoid areas of the intestine are often prominent, the cloacal bursa may be severely inflamed and characteristic haemorrhages are often present in the wall of the oesophagus. It should be stressed that haemorrhages may occur in any part of the digestive tract and also that free blood may fill the interior of the intestine or may be present in the abdominal cavity.

In birds which have survived the initial stages of the disease, haemorrhages in the oesophagus tend to heal and become replaced by surface scabs which become confluent, giving the appearance of a yellowish membrane adhering to the interior of the oesophagus.

The lesions described are so characteristic that a positive diagnosis can usually be made from them, although the precise post mortem picture depends on the age of bird affected, virulence of the infecting virus and degree of resistance of the flock. Where necessary virus isolation in the laboratory can be used to confirm diagnosis.

Treatment and Control

No treatment is of any value for duck virus enteritis. Hygiene measures give some degree of control, particularly prevention of spread of infection by keeping birds away from pond, or other water sources. A vaccine exists in the Netherlands and America for prevention of the disease. It is administered by subcutaneous innoculation to birds of two weeks of age or over and appears to give a reasonable degree of protection.

AVIAN INFLUENZA AND FOWL PLAGUE

Nature and Incidence

The term **avian influenza** refers to clinical infection by any of a large number of strains of influenza A virus. These give rise to a variety of disease syndromes in many countries, outbreaks usually being sporadic and involving respiratory signs. One of the most virulent of these infections and the best known of the influenza group of diseases is **fowl plague**; this occurs in chickens, turkeys, ducks and other bird species including many wild birds. The disease bears a strong resemblance to severe Newcastle disease and some confusion has existed in the U.K. as to the relationship between the two diseases, particularly since both have been referred to as fowl pest. In fact the two are caused by separate viruses and should be clearly differentiated as two distinct diseases. Fowl plague is now rarely diagnosed although less virulent types of avian influenza occur in many countries. However, a case of fowl plague, or a fowl plague-like disease, occurred in turkeys in eastern England in the Spring of 1979. This was the first recorded outbreak in Britain since 1963. The reasons for the sporadic occurrence of fowl plague are unknown, but wild birds are believed to act as an important means of transmission.

Signs

Signs of fowl plague resemble those of Newcastle disease and can be as variable. They include inappetance, dejection, coughing, nasal and ocular discharge, swollen sinuses and oedematous swelling of the head, diarrhoea and nervous signs. In some cases birds are found dead with no previous signs. Mortality rates vary from less than 10 per cent to over 50 per cent.

Post Mortem Changes

Post mortem changes are equally variable. There is often reddening of, and haemorrhages in, the skin, comb and wattles. Necrotic foci may be found in the liver, spleen, kidneys or other organs, and there may be thickening of the air sacs with fibrinous pericarditis and egg-peritonitis in laying birds.

It is not possible to distinguish between fowl plague and Newcastle disease on clinical signs or post mortem changes. These should, however, give rise to suspicion of one or other disease and confirmation depends on virus isolation by specialised laboratory techniques.

Spread and control

It is important that a differential diagnosis between the two diseases is made as rapidly as possible, not least because **fowl**

plague in the U.K. is still subject to a slaughter policy with compensation. This method of control has been abandoned in the case of Newcastle disease. It appears that close contact is necessary for spread of the virus and immediate slaughter and disposal of carcases is an effective method of prevention of spread and control of fowl plague. No spread to other flocks has taken place in the few cases of the disease which have occurred in Britain, following implementation of the slaughter policy. No other method of treatment or control of the disease is of any value and since wild birds are apparently the main source of infection it is doubtful if preventive measures could be made effective. The slaughter policy following diagnosis of the disease is clearly the best method of control.

HAEMORRHAGIC ENTERITIS OF TURKEYS

Nature and Course of Disease

This is an acute disease of turkeys which is of some importance in certain states of America and has recently (1978) occurred in two turkey flocks in Southern England.

The disease is caused by a virus and occurs mainly in turkeys of eight to twelve weeks.

Bird to bird transmission is by ingestion of virus in contaminated food or water, or from other contaminated sources. Signs include depression, listlessness, inappetance and blood in the droppings, or blood staining of the vent feathers. In many cases, however the first indication of the disease is sudden mortality, other signs only becoming evident after careful observation of the flock.

Post Mortem Changes and Diagnosis

The main post mortem findings are in the intestine and consist of extensive enteritis particularly of the duodenum or first part of the small intestine, with blood-stained fluid in the cavity of the gut. Haemorrhages may be found in the mucosa of the proventriculus and gizzard. Other changes include muscular haemorrhages, swelling and congestion of the liver, spleen, lungs and kidneys. A rather characteristic finding in the British cases was a marbled appearance of the cut surface of the spleen.

Diagnosis can generally be made from the signs and post mortem changes. Histological examination of various tissues may show inclusion bodies, and electron microscopy of spleens may reveal individual virus particles. The last mentioned investigation can as a rule be undertaken only by a specialised research laboratory.

Treatment

There is no useful treatment for haemorrhagic enteritis. Rigorous hygiene precautions may lessen the likelihood of introduction of infection from external sources.

CHAPTER 24

Diseases Caused by Fungi

Fungal diseases occur in poultry as in other animals, although the number of such infections is very much less than those caused by bacteria and viruses. In poultry, only three clearly defined fungal diseases are worthy of consideration. These are:

1. **Aspergillosis**
2. **Moniliasis**
3. **Favus.**

However, there is a good deal of evidence that a number of vaguely defined conditions occur which give rise to few visible clinical signs or post mortem changes but which adversely affect performance in affected flocks. Recent evidence points to the involvement of fungal infections in these cases and it is likely that as research work progresses the nature of these conditions will become clearer and fungi may be shown to have a greater causative role than was previously suspected.

It is now known that in addition to actual infection by fungal elements there exists a group of diseases which are caused not by fungi as such but by the toxic metabolites of fungi which have infected and multiplied in feed grains, other feed constituents or litter. It is important to distinguish between actual fungal infections in which the causative fungus invades the tissues, and those diseases due to ingestion by birds of toxic fungal metabolites in feed or litter. Such diseases are in effect a form of poising and are known collectively as mycotoxicoses. They are considered elsewhere.

ASPERGILLOSIS

This condition is due to invasion of the air passages, lungs and air sacs by the fungus *Aspergillus fumigatus*. It occurs in chickens, turkeys, game birds, pigeons and many other species and is of greatest economic importance in young chicks and turkey poults.

Aspergillus fumigatus and other fungi causing disease in poultry resemble in many ways those harmless fungi found on such materials as stale bread. They consist of a mass of fluffy filaments and reproduce by forming microscopic spores which are scattered throughout the environment, where they grow into fresh areas of mould. *Aspergillus fumigatus* is widely distributed in nature and grain, straw and similar materials stored in damp, warm conditions, can be a potent source of fungal spores.

Source of Infection

Aspergillosis occurs in **three fairly distinct age groups** in poultry and the source of infection tends to be different in these groups.

Baby Chicks

The disease is most commonly seen in baby chicks in the **first week of life** when it is often referred to as **brooder pneumonia**. In these cases, the disease is most commonly derived from the hatchery. Aspergillus is widely distributed in nature and contamination of egg-shells occurs readily, particularly where nest boxes are not kept clean, where eggs are not collected often enough or where eggs are laid on the floor of the breeding-house. The fungal spores then readily penetrate the shell; if such infected eggs are incubated, the fungus grows within the egg and at some stage of incubation one or two eggs may burst, and give rise to widespread distribution of spores within the incubator. The infection is thus transmitted to other chicks as they hatch, when they are most vulnerable to Aspergillosis infection by inhalation of fungal spores. Prevention of infection of eggs by the spores and avoidance of setting infected eggs is thus of the utmost importance.

Older Chicks

Aspergillosis is also encountered in slightly older chicks and poults, generally between **two and six weeks of age** . In these cases, the hatchery is seldom the source of infection, due to the interval of time elapsing between hatching and the first signs of disease in the flock. The source of infection can usually be traced to some form of

145

environmental contamination with mould. Often, particularly with turkey poults, it will be found that straw used as litter material has been damp, either at harvesting or during storage, giving ideal conditions for mould growth. If a bale of suspect straw is opened and shaken, clouds of dust will be seen arising from the straw; this dust may consist largely of vast numbers of fungal spores, inhalation of which will enable the fungus to develop in the birds' respiratory system.

Adult Birds

The third age group in which aspergillosis occurs is in adult birds. In these cases, however, only a single bird may be affected and this is often an aged member of a small backyard flock. The condition is not commonly seen in commercial flocks in the present modern poultry industry.

Aspergillosis in adult birds is a chronic condition so that the source of infection is often difficult or impossible to define. Many weeks may have passed between infection and diagnosis of Aspergillosis. However, at some previous stage the bird will have encountered a mould source and inhaled spores in the same manner as that described for younger birds.

Signs

Baby chicks suffering from aspergillosis lack vigour, have decreased appetite and, as the disease progresses, become very weak and emaciated. One of the most characteristic signs is a completely silent gaping or gasping, although in some cases coughing and rapid, difficult breathing may be more evident. In highly acute cases chicks may die very rapidly with few ante mortem signs.

In older chicks and poults, coughing and difficult breathing are usually evident with poor appetite, ruffled feathers, weakness and emaciation. In these birds the eyes are sometimes affected, cheesy accretions forming under the lids. Death may follow in a few days or a slow recovery with prolonged loss of condition may ensue.

In adult birds, the disease runs a chronic course with progressive emaciation and possibly some difficulty in breathing being the only noticeable signs. Death eventually occurs or the bird may be culled from the flock. Milder forms of the disease may occur in which few outward signs of ill-health are noted.

Post Mortem Findings

Post mortem examination of baby chicks or poults dying from

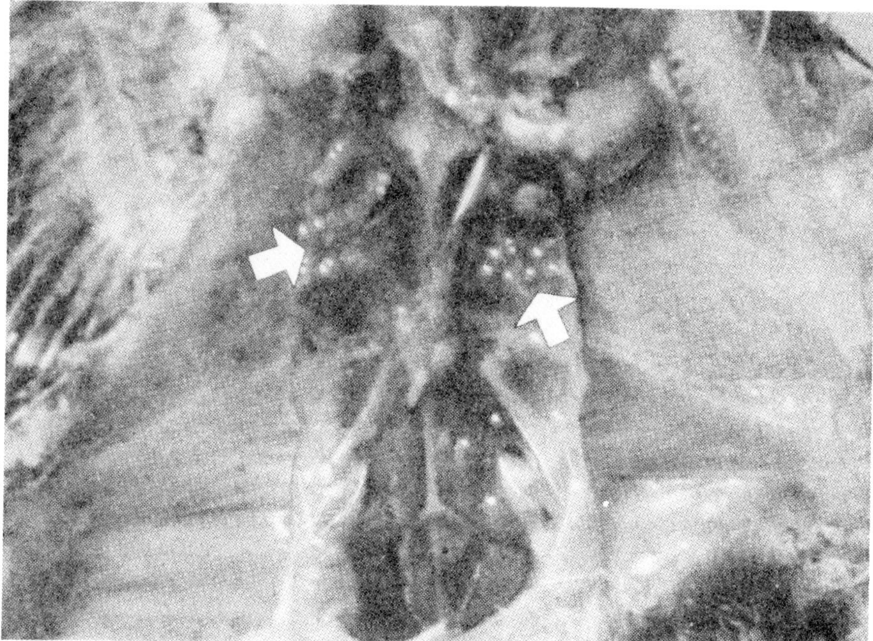

24.1   Aspergillosis involving the lungs of a turkey poult. White nodules of diseased tissue, indicated by the arrows, are scattered throughout the lungs.

acute aspergillosis shows changes in the lungs and air sacs, particularly multiple, yellow-white pin-head sized nodules scattered throughout the lung tissue. Lesions in air sacs may be similar or they may be small circular plaques with flat or concave surfaces. Sometimes coalescence of these lesions occurs with extensive involvement of air sacs and other organs. Occasionally plaques of yellow caseous material are found under the eyelids or in the facial sinuses. It should be noted that in many cases the lesions of aspergillosis in young chicks are extremely minute and can be overlooked unless a very careful examination is made.

In older birds, lesions take the form of grey-white solid masses in the lungs which rapidly form large irregular nodules sometimes almost totally replacing the lung tissue. Plaque-like lesions may occur in the air sacs and sometimes cotton-wool like fungal masses are grossly visible. Frequently the bronchi and lower trachea are also invaded. In adult birds, the commonest lesions are single or multiple, blue-green furry masses in the air sacs; sometimes these become so extensive as almost to occlude the air sacs. These lesions are so characteristic that they are unlikely to be confused with any other condition. As the fungal growth spreads, other abdominal organs may become involved including the intestines, liver and kidneys. In some cases extensive adhesions between these organs are found.

Diagnosis

The lesions of aspergillosis are rather characteristic and should give rise to suspicion of the disease on post mortem examination provided a careful inspection of the lungs is made. Confirmation of the diagnosis is easily achieved in the laboratory by culture of the fungus on **Sabourauds medium.** The fungus grows readily on this special medium, blue-green furry masses usually appearing after two days incubation.

Treatment and Prevention

There is **no satisfactory treatment** for affected birds. Anti-bacterial antibiotics are of no value and even anti-fungal antibiotics apparently have little effect on this condition. **Affected birds should be destroyed.**

Prevention of the condition in baby chicks requires the same precautions regarding cleanliness of hatching eggs and incubation hygiene as were discussed in the chapter on yolk sac infection. Hatching eggs should be collected as frequently as possible, nest boxes must be clean and floor-laid eggs rejected for hatching. Incubation should begin as soon as possible after eggs are laid and the highest possible standards of hygiene at the hatchery should be maintained at all times. Eggs intended for hatching should be **fumigated with formaldehyde** as soon as possible after collection and if necessary again on arrival at the hatchery before incubation.

In older chicks and poults, infection is usually acquired by inhalation of spores from a mould source, frequently musty straw. The use of straw for turkey litter is inadvisable due to its frequent incrimination in outbreaks of aspergillosis.

If it is shown that straw is not the source or if an outbreak of Aspergillosis occurs where straw is not being used then another source of mould, such as stale food, must be sought. Once identified, the source must be removed and replaced, or the birds moved to fresh premises. When this is done it is often surprising how quickly losses stop and the flock recovers.

In sporadic cases in adult birds it is usually difficult to locate the mould source and little can be done other than culling of affected birds.

MONILIASIS

Moniliasis, or thrush, as it is sometimes called is caused by the fungus *Monilia albicans* or *Candida albicans*. It occurs in chickens, turkeys and several kinds of game birds. Although the disease is not of great consequence, several serious outbreaks have occurred in Britain, principally in young turkeys.

The causal agent is frequently found in small numbers in the gut of healthy animals where it causes no apparent harm, but, under certain conditions, it may multiply enormously.

Signs

Moniliasis does not produce characteristic signs of ill-health and, when it is associated with other diseases, it is naturally difficult to decide which are responsible for the particular signs observed. But, in general, affected turkey poults and chicks have a thoroughly dejected appearance, the feathers are rough, the appetite poor and growth rate slow or non-existent. The disease may terminate in death, particularly in very young birds.

Post Mortem Findings

At post mortem examination, the most striking changes are found in the crop, the inner surface of which is covered with a thick, whitish material which piles up, giving the appearance of turkish towelling. This material can easily be scraped off to expose the inflamed wall of the crop which may be covered with ulcers. The crop itself usually contains thick, slimy, sour-smelling fluid.

Prevention and Control

As regards treatment, the suitability of the diet should be considered, and also hygiene, sanitation and the possibility of over-crowding. If any other disease co-exists in the affected group of birds, immediate corrective measures should be implemented.

Some authorities recommend adding chemicals such as copper sulphate to the drinking water, but general agreement does not exist as to their efficacy. Others recommend the addition to the food of an anti-fungal antibiotic called nystatin at a level of 50 grams per ton for several weeks.

FAVUS

Favus is a chronic disease of the skin caused by a fungus called

Trichophyton gallinae. It affects poultry, principally chickens and turkeys, and also other animals and man. It has been reported in many parts of the world and is said to be not uncommon in France, but it is classed in Britain as a rare disease.

Signs

Favus is characterised by the development of white powdery-like spots on the unfeathered parts of the head. As the disease progresses the spots enlarge and join together to form wrinkled crusts or scabs.

In severe cases, the infection also involves the feathered parts of the body and as a consequence the feathers fall out in patches, the exposed skin becoming thickened and crusty. Severely affected birds may show considerable loss of condition and become weak and anaemic. The disease spreads throughout a flock by direct contact.

In the laboratory, the causative fungus can be isolated by prolonged culture (up to four weeks) on Sabourauds medium of material removed from a lesion.

Prevention and Control

Badly affected birds should be killed and those mildly affected should be segregated. If it is considered worthwhile treating the condition, removal of crusts with soap and water, and application of an ointment consisting of 5 per cent formalin in petroleum jelly appears to be effective. Since **human beings can become infected,** care should be taken in handling diseased birds.

CHAPTER 25

Coccidiosis

THREAT TO MODERN POULTRY INDUSTRY

Coccidiosis is probably the most prevalent and certainly one of the most serious infectious diseases of poultry. It has a world-wide distribution occurring wherever poultry are reared. It is commonest in chickens but severe outbreaks in turkey flocks are also common; ducks and geese are occasionally affected.

Most chickens come into contact with the disease sometime during their life, although the great majority show no signs of ill-health. Young, closely confined birds are mainly affected and it is no exaggeration to say that were it not for timely research into the disease, which has resulted in the development of effective preventive and curative products, present methods of keeping poultry under intensive systems would never have become a practical proposition. Even now, in spite of widespread use of these drugs severe outbreaks still occur and the disease remains one of the most serious threats to the poultry industry.

Cause

Coccidiosis in poultry is a disease of the intestines caused by microscopic parasitic organisms (*protozoa*) called *coccidia*. A number of different genera exist within the protozoan group, and cause the disease in various animal species, including pigs, calves and dogs. In these species, however, the disease is relatively uncommon in comparison with the situation in poultry, although it is also common in rabbits. In poultry, coccidiosis is caused by various species of the genus *Eimeria*, each species causing disease in only one type of bird. *Eimeria tenella*, for example, infects only chickens and

151

E.adenoides infects only turkeys. Thus the coccidia are said to be **host specific** and therefore it can be stated quite emphatically that coccidiosis of the chicken will not spread to turkeys, nor will rabbit coccidiosis infect chickens. This rule can be applied to all types of coccidiosis and any animal species, in marked contrast to diseases such as blackhead which will readily spread from chickens to turkeys.

Several types

At least eight different types of coccidiosis occur in chickens and at least seven in turkeys. It should be pointed out, however, that although some of these types may, under certain conditions, produce severe disease, others are relatively harmless.

With few exceptions, the different kinds of coccidia parasitise the intestines of animals and birds. One exception is a coccidium of geese, *E.truncata*, in which the kidneys are the site of infection.

Development cycle

Coccidia undergo a very complicated cycle of development both within and outside the animal body, the cycle being essentially the same irrespective of the kind of coccidium involved. The stage in the cycle at which the disease is transmitted from bird to bird is called the **oocyst**. Oocysts are passed in the droppings of infected birds and on the ground they undergo a process of "ripening" called **sporulation.** Only after this process is completed are they capable of setting up the disease if swallowed by a susceptible bird. Sporulation takes a variable time, but it is rarely less than two days, depending largely on environmental conditions. It occurs most rapidly under moist warm conditions and most slowly under dry cold conditions. Oocysts are extremely resistant forms and may survive outside the body for as long as eighteen months. They are **not killed by commonly used disinfectants**, and it is a mistake to believe that dipping of boots in a disinfectant solution before entering a poultry house will prevent mechanical transmission of coccidiosis.

Sporulated occysts, when swallowed by susceptible birds undergo further development and eventually disintegrate liberating new forms called sporozoites which penetrate the cells lining the gut. The sporozoites develop into further stages called schizonts which undergo further development and liberate large numbers of new stages called merozoites. This is the stage of asexual reproduction or schizogony and it may be repeated two or three times with formation of additional schizonts and merozoites at each asexual cycle.

Following the asexual phase, a further process of sexual reproduction occurs with formation of male and female gametocytes which unite to form oocysts. When these are passed in the droppings the life cycle is complete. It will be seen that a moderate intake of sporulated oocysts may result in extremely heavy oocyst elimination in the droppings, with a rapid build up of oocysts in the litter from which the bird readily re-infects itself. If the bird is **prevented from ingesting oocysts from droppings, or if conditions for sporulation are unfavourable** the likelihood of a coccidiosis outbreak is reduced. It is mainly because birds in cages have little access to their droppings, and hence limited oocyst intake, that coccidiosis is seldom seen in cage reared birds. In birds on litter where moist, warm conditions prevail and where birds are over-crowded, coccidiosis is likely to break out. Most birds develop sub-clinical infections with small numbers of oocysts being continually passed into the litter from which they re-infect themselves and infect other birds. This continuous low level intake of oocysts stimulates immunity in the bird or flock with no evidence of disease. If on the other hand, very large numbers are ingested over a short period of time the massive invasion of the gut that results may give rise to such severe damage that rapid death occurs. Avoidance of over-crowding, together with correct litter maintenance, particularly prevention of wet patches around drinkers, will help to prevent outbreaks of coccidiosis.

The length of the coccidial life cycle varies from about four to seven days depending on the type of coccidium involved, and the environmental conditions.

TWO MAIN TYPES OF COCCIDIOSIS IN CHICKENS

Caecal Coccidiosis

This is one of the most severe forms of coccidiosis and is caused by *Eimeria tenella*. It is also one of the commonest forms of the disease and practically all chickens will become infected at some time during their lives. Whether they show signs depends on the level of disease challenge, that is, on the number of oocysts they pick up and the rapidity of their ingestion.

The disease occurs typically at about four weeks of age but outbreaks may be seen earlier or later. The standard case shows dullness, loss of weight and blood in the droppings. There is inappetance and affected birds stand apart from the flock with closed eyes and ruffled feathers. In severe untreated outbreaks there may be rapid death of many birds and mortality may reach 95 per cent. Although blood in the droppings is often mentioned as a typical finding in caecal coccidiosis, this is unlikely to be the first sign of the disease noticed by the poultry farmer. Only a small number of birds are likely to be affected at one time so that only a few droppings contain blood. In the reduced light of the modern poultry house these are unlikely to be noticed and it is more likely that the first sign of the disease noticed by the owner will be a few birds looking depressed and off their food.

Post mortem changes and diagnosis

Post mortem of a severe case shows enlarged and inflamed caecal tubes distended by blood from haemorrhages due to widespread erosion of the caecal mucous membrane. In some more chronic cases the caecal walls may be thickened and fibrosed and the caecal tubes contain cores of creamy brown caseous material. These must be distinguished from the cores of blackhead and it should be borne in mind that the latter disease does occasionally occur in chickens.

Diagnosis is usually easily confirmed from post mortem findings. Vast numbers of oocysts are seen microscopically in smears from caecal mucous membrane, or, if the bird examined is in the early stage of the disease, schizonts and merozoites may be seen.

Intestinal Coccidiosis

A number of different species of *Eimeria* may cause intestinal coccidiosis, some kinds being more harmful than others. Many outbreaks are due to mixed infection by two or more *Eimeria* species, the pathogenic effects depending on the predominating species. However *E. necatrix* is the most pathogenic type and others of importance are *E. acervulina*, *E. maxima* and *E. brunetti*. A short description of the effects of each type of intestinal coccidiosis is given in the following paragraphs. The commonest species are undoubtedly *E. necatrix* and *E. acervulina* although in many cases of coccidiosis the precise species involved is not easily identified.

Eimeria necatrix

This species causes the most severe intestinal coccidiosis in chick-

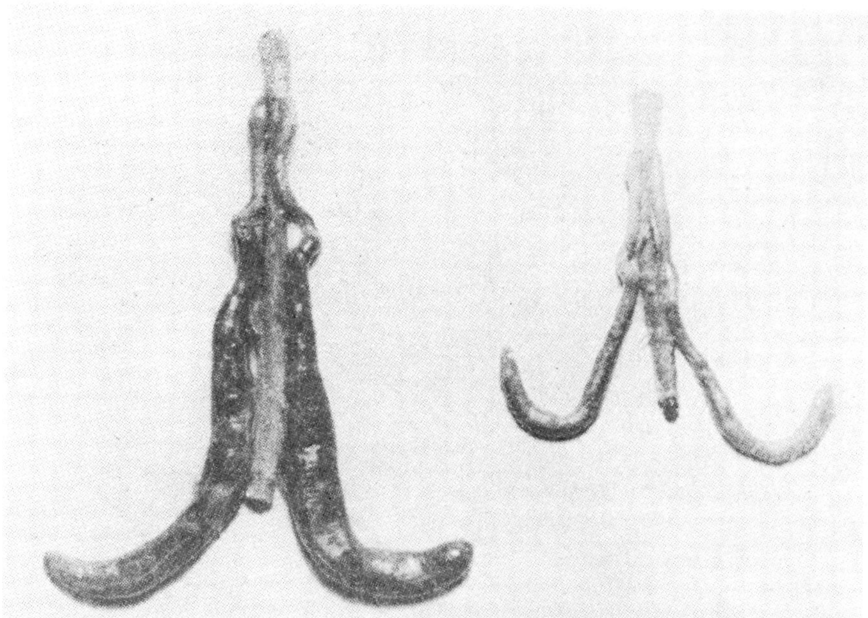

25.1 Diseased (left) and healthy caecal tubes. The degree of inflammation depends upon the severity of the attack of coccidiosis.

ens. Outbreaks occur usually in birds over six weeks of age and may be seen in maturing pullets or even occasionally in birds in lay. Affected birds are dejected, off their food and lose weight. Diarrhoea may be present but generally there is no blood in the droppings. In untreated cases, mortality can be high although spread is usually slower than in caecal coccidiosis.

On **post mortem** examination the middle portion of the small intestine is found to be affected. There is often severe distension of the bowel, thickening of the bowel wall with haemorrhage into the gut from erosion of the mucous membrane. The intestinal content often consists of a mass of blood-stained mucus, and haemorrhages and white spots are seen in the bowel wall. Microscopic examination of smears from the affected region of the intestine shows groups of large schizonts. No oocysts are found in the affected area; in this particular type of coccidiosis oocysts are produced in the caeca. In other respects, however, the caeca are normal and there should be no confusion between this type of coccidiosis and caecal coccidiosis due to *E.tenella*.

Blood in the droppings, it should be emphasised, is not a common feature of *E.necatrix* infection and it should be said that this occurs commonly only in *E.tenella* infection. It is a common mistake to believe that blood is seen in droppings in all coccidiosis infections; in fact it occurs in only a minority of cases.

Eimeria acervulina

This type of coccidiosis is rather common but it does not cause heavy mortality. The effects tend to be mild depression, reduced appetite and reduced weight gain although in severe infections a few birds may die. The condition is usually seen in replacement birds in the late rearing stages or in early lay.

Post mortem changes are usually found in the duodenum, the upper part of the small intestine. White spots or streaks are visible on the external surface of the bowel. The internal lining is slightly thickened and reddened and the intestinal content is a pink or cream coloured mucus. Severe inflammation of the bowel however is not a feature and no blood is present in the bowel. In some cases the changes are so slight that they may be easily missed unless the gut is carefully examined.

Microscopic examination of intestinal smears shows the presence of vast numbers of oocysts. *E.acervulina* is one of the most prolific oocyst producers of all coccidial species although it produces less severe disease than a number of other types.

Eimeria maxima

This type of coccidiosis attacks the middle portion of the bowel and can be responsible for significant mortality, usually in birds over six weeks old. Affected birds are depressed, appetite is lost and a watery white diarrhoea develops.

The post mortem changes resemble those of *E.necatrix* although they are generally less severe. The mid gut is distended, the walls thickened and in heavy infections there may be haemorrhage into the intestine. Microscopic examination of intestinal smears shows the characteristic large oocysts. The oocysts of this species are larger than those of any other type of coccidiosis affecting poultry.

Eimeria praecox

This species also affects the upper intestine and its effects are similar to those of *E. acervulina*. Only mild disease is usually caused, with some inappetance and weight loss. Mortality is low or negligible.

Eimeria brunetti

This species affects the lower half of the small intestine and the large intestine. Mortality is variable but in severe infections it can be high. Numerous haemorrhages are present in the lower bowel wall and there is blood stained mucus in the intestine. There may also be some blood in the droppings. Microscopic examination of a smear from the lower intestine shows rounded oocysts of variable size.

Diagnosis

Diagnosis of coccidiosis can, in most cases, be made from a consideration of clinical signs, microscopic examination of intestinal smears, and post mortem changes. In mild cases, careful examination is required to detect lesions and in all cases the entire length of the bowel should be examined. The type of coccidiosis present can often be accurately diagnosed from the appearance of the lesions and the region of the bowel affected. In some cases the size and shape of the oocysts or the presence of other stages, such as schizonts in *E.necatrix* infection, can be helpful. In other coccidiosis outbreaks the species cannot easily be identified on routine post mortem examination. However, it is not always essential to identify the species; rapid diagnosis and immediate treatment are the objectives when dealing with coccidiosis.

It should be said that in some cases a few oocysts may be found in intestinal smears in the absence of clinical signs or lesions. These cases have been called coccidiasis but it is a **mistake to diagnose coccidiosis on the single finding of a small number of oocysts.** However a careful watch should be kept on such flocks, as a build-up of oocyst levels may occur with clinical disease following later.

Another possible pitfall in diagnosis of coccidiosis involves the bacterial infection **necrotic enteritis.** This infection sometimes follows coccidiosis and, although the lesions are somewhat different, the two diseases may be confused. In cases of poor response to coccidiosis treatment it should be ensured that the reason is not the presence of necrotic enteritis. Where it is, immediate treatment with penicillin should be commenced.

Treatment

Effective anticoccidial drugs are available for treatment of the disease. Most modern preparations contain one or more of the **sulphonamide** drugs. Originally sulphadimidine was used but the most commonly used drug at present is **sulphaquinoxaline.** To be effective, treatment must be started as soon as possible after a diagnosis is made. The usual method of medication is addition of the drug to the drinking water, and where sulphonamides are used the course is normally three days medicated water followed by two days off treatment and another three days medication. In many cases this is sufficient to effect a cure but if the flock has not totally recovered another three day course following a second two day break may be necessary.

Other preparations available contain a combination of non-sulphonamide drugs, such as **amprolium** and **ethopabate.** A number of anticoccidial preparations contain a sulphonamide, usually sulphaquinoxaline, together with another drug such as **diaveridine.** The two drugs potentiate each other, that is to say, their combined effect is greater than the added effects of the two drugs acting separately. Any of the modern anticoccidial preparations are effective and their use generally results in a rapid cure. In cases where response is less than anticipated the reason may be incorrect dilution of the drug, treatment started too late in the course of the disease or the presence of other disease in the flock in addition to coccidiosis.

It should be borne in mind that **sulphonamides adversely affect hatchability** of eggs, and for this reason, where it is necessary to treat breeding birds which are in production, a treatment other than sulphonamide should be used.

PREVENTION AND CONTROL

The modern poultry industry has come to rely heavily on anti-coccidial drugs, or **coccidiostats** as they are usually called, incorporated in the food for prevention of coccidiosis. Indeed, it is sometimes forgotten that these substances are an **adjunct to good management rather than a substitute** for it. Sound management practices will go a long way towards prevention of coccidiosis, the aim being to allow exposure of the bird to small numbers of oocysts so that immunity is developed to the disease, but to prevent oocyst numbers building up to a stage where clinical disease results. In theory this could be achieved by removing birds' droppings every two days, thus preventing intake of significant numbers of sporulated oocysts (only "ripe" or sporulated oocysts can initiate the disease when swallowed by the bird). In practice, of course, this is impossible, but efficient hygiene measures, cleanliness, avoidance of overcrowding, maintaining stock in good health and free from other diseases, adequate nutrition, correct litter management and, above all, avoidance of wet patches in litter are commonsense measures which help to prevent the disease. Unfortunately, such management ideals are not always achieved under farm conditions and it has become almost universal practice to supplement the feeds of rearing birds with coccidiostats as an aid to prevention of coccidiosis. It should be appreciated however that coccidiostats control the disease only up to a certain level of challenge, and when this is exceeded an outbreak can occur in spite of the presence of the coccidiostat at the correct inclusion level. Hence the need for good management practices in addition to use of coccidiostats.

Over the years, a great many coccidiostats have been developed and marketed, some achieving more success than others. New compounds continue to be added to the market, at enormous expense to the drug houses since stringent tests of safety and efficacy are required before a new coccidiostat is cleared for use. One of the most successful in recent years has been **monensin** which has captured a very large share of the broiler coccidiostat market in the U.K. and elsewhere. Probably the most commonly used coccidiostat for pullet flocks is a combination of sulpha-quinoxaline, amprolium and ethopabate.

Prevention in broilers

The aim of coccidiostat inclusion in broiler rations is total suppression of the disease throughout the life of the flock, and so successful have coccidiostats become that coccidiosis is now only occasionally encountered in broilers, although it is still a potential threat to the broiler industry. Usually when cases occur the reason can be found in incorrect inclusion levels, other disease affecting the birds resulting in reduced food and coccidiostat intake, poor management with wet patches around drinkers and so on. A factor which must be considered, however, is the possibility of a particular species of *Eimeria* developing resistance to a particular coccidiostat and this should always be considered in coccidiosis outbreaks in broilers.

It should be noted that a number of broiler coccidiostats are subject to a withdrawal period i.e. the drug must be withdrawn from feed at a stated time, usually three days, before the flock is killed. This prevents the possibility of the presence of tissue residues in the marketed bird which might be harmful to the consumer.

Prevention in Pullets

In the case of pullets, the aim of coccidiostat inclusion is not total suppression of the disease as in broilers, but prevention of clinical disease, at the same time allowing the life cycle of the organism to develop to a stage where it stimulates an immune response on the part of the bird. Were such immunity not achieved, pullets would be totally susceptible to coccidiosis on withdrawal of the drug before lay, with potentially catastrophic results. It is the necessity to allow development of immunity which makes the use of coccidiostats less effective in pullets than in broilers. Indeed, many of the highly effective broiler coccidiostats are not licensed for use in the feed of pullets. These and other factors such as the smaller appetites of pullets and the use of interrupted or restricted feed programmes, which may reduce coccidiostat intake, result in coccidiosis being much more commonly encountered in pullets than in broilers. It should also be remembered that certain coccidial species are less susceptible than others to the action of coccidiostats. For example *E.acervulina* is much less effectively controlled than *E.tenella* or *E.necatrix*.

Post-outbreak measures

There are two schools of thought regarding the action to be taken by way of disinfection of a poultry house following an outbreak of coccidiosis. Some authorities suggest that the house should be thoroughly cleaned of all litter, dust and cobwebs, washed out with water and disinfected by spraying a solution of ammonia which is lethal to oocysts. Others are of the opinion that such thorough cleaning of the house is unnecessary. They say that the litter may be left in the house, the new chicks thus meeting the infection early in life, so ensuring a rapid immune response to the disease and rendering a clinical outbreak less likely. There is no doubt that many severe coccidiosis outbreaks have occurred in new poultry houses where birds have not been reared before. It must be accepted that it is virtually impossible to rear birds free from coccidia and even in a clean house oocysts will make their appearance, with the possibility of severe disease if conditions are right for a rapid build-up and the flock has no previously developed immunity. In cases where it is decided not to change the litter between crops of birds, the litter should at least be heaped and allowed to heat. The temperature reached by this process is sufficient to kill a majority of the oocysts, a small number surviving to give rise to early immunity in the next flock. The resistance of oocysts to the

160

commonly used disinfectants and to formaldehyde fumigation is again emphasised. Only **ammonia** and the gas **methyl bromide** will effectively kill oocysts, but these substances are so unpleasant and dangerous to human operators that they are seldom used under practical conditions.

It is probably true to say that whether or not a poultry house is thoroughly cleaned out, the next flock is at risk from coccidiosis, and that avoidance of clinical disease depends on the skill of the stockman aided by suppression of the parasite by coccidiostats.

COCCIDIOSIS IN TURKEYS

Coccidiosis in turkeys is becoming an increasing problem in intensively managed turkey flocks. Eight or nine coccidial types have been reported from turkeys but only three or, possibly, four cause clinical disease, the others being non-pathogenic. The species which gives rise to the most serious disease is *E.adenoides* which affects the lower small intestine and caeca. Also important is *E.meleagrimitis* in the upper intestine. *E.gallopavonis* and *E.meleagridis* may cause disease of the rectum and caeca respectively although the latter is often regarded as being harmless.

The signs of coccidiosis in turkeys are similar to those described in chickens except that blood rarely appears in the droppings. Instead there is often a white slimy diarrhoea and there tends to be a characteristic smell in a poultry house in which many affected poults are present. The disease is often seen at a younger age in poults than in chicks, sometimes as early as ten days of age. In turkeys however a true age-immunity appears to develop, the disease being rarely if ever seen in birds over ten weeks of age.

An outbreak in turkey poults may occur extremely suddenly — up to 15 per cent of the birds may die overnight. Many others show typical signs of huddling, ruffled feathers, standing with eyes closed and loud cheeping. The disease is diagnosed in the same way as in chickens, but haemorrhagic bowel lesions are less frequent. Instead a creamy mucoid material is found in the intestines and in the caeca; it sometimes forms into a caseous plug in the caecal tubes. Occasionally the upper bowel wall shows haemorrhages in *E.meleagrimitis* infection.

Microscopic examination of intestinal or caecal smears shows in most cases vast numbers of oocysts. It should be remembered that non-pathogenic coccidial types occur in turkeys so that simply finding oocysts does not confirm the disease. However, a combination of clinical signs, post mortem changes and presence of large numbers of oocysts is sufficient evidence on which to base a diagnosis and commence treatment.

Turkeys tend to be more fastidious in their drinking habits than chickens and are often reluctant to drink anything other than pure water. It is usually found that sulphaquinoxaline medicated water is most readily accepted and it is wise to offer this rather than combinations of drugs. Sometimes dosing of affected birds by passing a tube through the mouth into the crop is worthwhile, particularly where small numbers of birds are involved. This is a simple technique which can be learned by the average stockman in a matter of minutes.

The principles of prevention and control are the same for turkeys as for broiler chickens. Coccidiostats are used in the feed but some of the most effective ones are not licensed for use in turkeys. This and the turkey's apparent lack of "will to live" when compared with chickens may help to explain the higher incidence and mortality from coccidiosis in turkey poults.

COCCIDIOSIS IN OTHER BIRDS

Coccidiosis does occur in **ducklings,** although only rarely in comparison with chickens and turkeys. The disease tends to occur as a sudden, explosive outbreak with high mortality in a short time. The type of coccidium usually involved is believed to be one known as *Tyzzeria perniciosa* and lesions occur in the small intestine, rather resembling those of *E.necatrix* infection in chickens. It is likely that as duck farming becomes more intensive, coccidiosis will increase in frequency and importance in this species.

The condition generally responds well to sulphaquinoxaline in the water, although the drinking habits of ducks makes water medication rather uncertain. Should coccidiosis occur in ducks on a pond, it is best to remove the birds from the pond and confine them to a pen where only medicated water is available, otherwise it is unlikely that they will consume sufficient medicated water to cure the disease.

Geese are affected by two types of coccidiosis one of which, *E.anseris,* causes disease of the small intestine resembling *E.necatrix* infection in chickens. The other, caused by *E.truncata,* is unusual in that it affects the kidneys rather than the intestine, although development of the parasite starts in the intestine. This is an important disease in certain European countries where large numbers of geese are reared. Goslings of three to twelve weeks are susceptible and mortality can be extremely high. Affected kidneys are swollen and mottled, and smears from kidneys examined microscopically show large numbers of oocysts.

Coccidiosis is an important disease of intensively reared **pheasants and partridges**. The condition is seen in poults from two weeks up to ten or twelve weeks of age and resembles coccidiosis in the turkey; the caeca are affected and creamy-coloured caseous deposits are usually visible in the caecal tubes. Mortality can be very high. Treatment with sulphaquinoxaline is usually successful although amprolium and ethopabate medicated water is sometimes more readily taken by game birds. It should be borne in mind that hexamitiasis is not uncommon in pheasants and in cases where response to treatment for coccidiosis is less than expected a check should be made for the presence of a complicating hexamitiasis infection.

CHAPTER 26

Blackhead

NATURE AND INCIDENCE

Blackhead is an acutely infectious disease of turkeys which, until recently, was one of the greatest menaces to successful rearing. Blackhead derives its name from the darkening of the head which is sometimes seen in affected birds. This is not a constant feature of the disease and the scientific name histomoniasis is to be preferred.

While the disease occurs mainly in turkeys, it has also been seen in pheasants, partridges, pea-fowl, grouse and some wild birds. The disease in chickens usually takes a mild form but some severe outbreaks have occurred, usually in association with intensive rearing methods. Despite this, it is still true to say that the main importance of blackhead in chickens is that it constitutes a prime source of infection for turkeys. It is well known that co-rearing of chickens and turkeys often results in the turkeys contracting blackhead.

Cause

Blackhead is caused by a microscopic parasite, a protozoan called *Histomonas meleagridis* or, more simply, "**the blackhead parasite**".

Spread

The causative organism occurs in the caecal tubes of affected birds where it multiplies enormously and passes out in the droppings; exposed to the atmosphere it dies in a matter of hours. For many years, early in the present century, researchers were unable to explain not only how the disease passed from bird to bird but also how ground could remain infectious for many months after removal of infected birds. Eventually it was shown that the extremely resistant eggs of the caecal worm, *Heterakis gallinae*, acted as carrier agents for the organism.

Development cycle

By some means as yet uncertain, the *Histomonad* organisms gain entry to the eggs of the caecal worm and later into the larvae which develop within the eggs. These eggs are then passed in the birds' droppings. Only *Histomonads* which gain entry to these eggs will infect poults when they are ingested; those which are passed in the droppings unprotected by the eggs will soon die or, even if they are quickly ingested by other poults, will be killed by the intestinal juices.

After the *Heterakis* eggs are passed in the droppings they undergo, on the ground, a period of development lasting seven to fourteen days, varying with the temperature and humidity. Eggs swallowed by turkeys after this development period hatch in the bird's intestine and the emerging *Heterakis* larvae rapidly move to the caeca, burrowing into its walls and causing the release of any *Histomonas* organisms that were contained in the eggs, and subsequently the larvae. These *Histomonads* multiply rapidly in the tissues of the caecal wall causing considerable damage in this area. Some of the organisms gain entry to the bloodstream and are carried to the liver where they produce the typical circular lesions in this organ. Others again infect *Heterakis* worm eggs, and are passed with these eggs in the droppings and so restart the cycle.

It is known that *Histomonas* organisms can survive in the eggs of *Heterakis gallinae* for long periods, possibly as long as the eggs themselves. Observations made under practical conditions indicate that turkeys put on land occupied many months previously by infected poultry will pick up the disease. Since chickens are commonly parasitised by *Heterakis* worms, some eggs of which frequently contain *Histomonas* organisms, it is apparent that the practice of rearing turkeys alongside chickens is fraught with hazard.

It has been shown that *Heterakis* eggs may be ingested by earthworms, inside which the larvae hatch out, and may live for long periods in the earthworm's tissues. If these eggs and larvae contain *Histomonas* organisms, eating of the earthworms by turkeys may result in an outbreak of the disease. This may be an important means of transmission of the disease in certain circumstances but generally the main means of transmission is ingestion of *Heterakis* eggs directly without the assistance of any other agent.

Signs

Turkey poults of from **one to three months of age are most susceptible** to blackhead, and it is in these that the heaviest losses occur. In untreated flocks of this age mortality rate may reach 70 to 90 per cent.

The first signs of the disease are depression and drowsiness, followed by loss of appetite and increased thirst. The birds are reluctant to move and stand around with feathers ruffled, wings drooping and head lowered. At a slightly later stage, diarrhoea becomes a feature and the droppings of some birds assume a characteristic sulphur-yellow colour. The earlier signs of depression become ever more marked and within a few days of signs being noticed the first deaths occur.

Older turkeys have a greater degree of resistance and in them the course of the disease is more prolonged, but may still be severe and a high proportion of these older birds may contract the infection. Affected birds appear unthrifty and suffer from a persistent diarrhoea. They become very thin and ultimately die or make a slow recovery. During this time their droppings constitute a potent source of infection for susceptible turkeys.

Post Mortem Findings

Histomonas meleagridis affects mainly the caeca and liver and the main post mortem changes are found in these organs. The caecal tubes are enlarged, the walls thickened and inflamed and they become filled with a mass of solid, caseous material. These caseous caecal "cores" tend to adhere to the caecal walls. Often the walls are severely damaged and ulcerated, and the ulcers may perforate and give rise to fatal peritonitis. The lesions on the liver consist of large, circular, slightly depressed, greyish-white or yellowish areas studded over its surface. They vary considerably in number from a few to being, in the later stages, so plentiful as to cover most of the liver surface.

These changes are rather characteristic of blackhead and when they are found along with the earlier mentioned signs, the disease should immediately be suspected. Absolute confirmation of diagnosis requires microscopic demonstration of the organism from caecal lesions, and for this birds must be delivered live to a diagnostic laboratory.

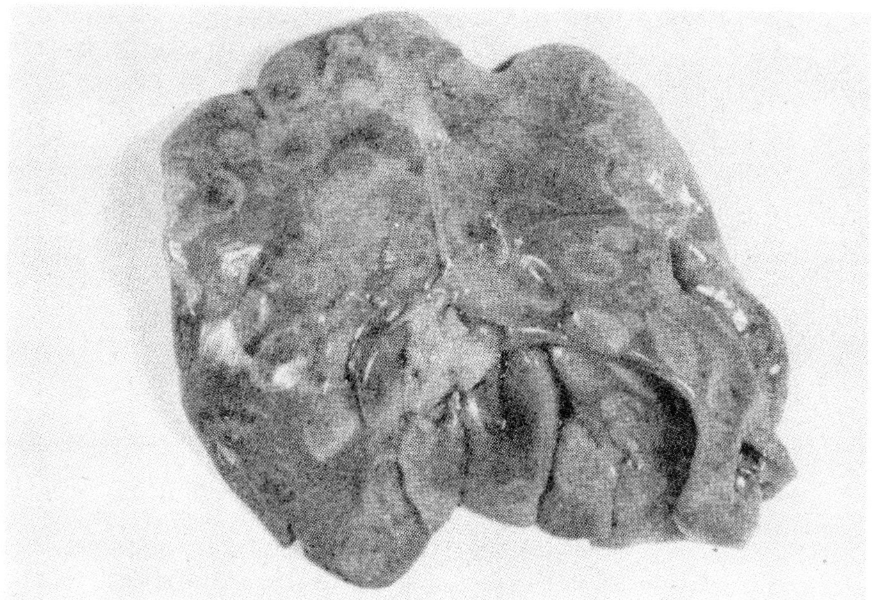

26.1 Liver from a turkey suffering with blackhead. The surface is studded with large greyish-white or yellow areas.

PREVENTION AND TREATMENT

Over the years many drugs have been used to treat blackhead some with more effect than others. Now the drug **dimetridazole** is commonly used for prevention and treatment. In order to prevent the disease the drug is included in the food at a rate of 0.0125 to 0.015 per cent and the medicated food given as long as birds are at risk. Other drugs used for prevention include **nifursol** and **furazolidone.**

Effective treatment of the disease is now possible by use of dimetridazole administered in the drinking water; it must be given early in the course of an outbreak and it should be noted that severely ill birds are unlikely to recover. Treatment must continue for ten days, when the outbreak should be under control, although relapses are liable to occur, because the birds are apparently unable to build up any immunity to the disease; the drug should, therefore, be kept in readiness to recommence treatment if necessary.

It should be emphasised that drug treatment of the disease must be regarded as a **supplement, rather than an alternative to good**

management and **high standards of hygiene**. Cases of blackhead are most likely to be seen under conditions in which the general health and management of the flock is poor and when exposure to infection is heavy.

Since blackhead is transmitted via the *Heterakis* egg, flock management should aim at reducing the risk of turkeys picking up the eggs. As already mentioned, chickens often harbour *Heterakis* worms and it is essential to **avoid contact between chickens and turkeys.** Worming of chickens and turkeys with a broad spectrum wormer will reduce the number of worms, and hence the number of eggs passed to contaminate the environment.

It is no doubt a reflection of the efficiency of preventive medication that the number of outbreaks of blackhead in turkeys is decreasing year by year. The fact that outbreaks do occur would seem to indicate that considerable numbers of *Heterakis* worms and their eggs containing *Histomonas* organisms are still present in the environment. There seems little hope at present that the disease will be eliminated or reduced to such low levels that preventive medication can be dispensed with in the foreseeable future.

CHAPTER 27

Hexamitiasis

NATURE AND INCIDENCE

Hexamitiasis is an infectious disease of turkeys caused by a protozoan called *Hexamita meleagridis*. Although not as economically important as blackhead it is responsible on occasion for serious losses in turkey flocks. The disease had been known for many years but it was not until 1938 that it was found to be due to a *Hexamita* organism. Although it was fairly common in this country in the nineteen-fifties its incidence has now been reduced and it must be described as a rare disease in turkeys in Britain at the present time. It does, however, occur in **pheasant** flocks and in these it can be responsible for severe losses; it is important to distinguish between hexamitiasis and coccidiosis in these birds. The disease does not occur in chickens, ducks or geese but outbreaks have been reported in partridge and quail.

The disease in turkeys occurs mainly in poults under twelve weeks of age; older birds in this age group do not usually contract the disease unless they are subjected to unfavourable management conditions and it is much less severe than in younger poults.

Source of Infection

Susceptible turkeys contract hexamitiasis by consuming food, water, soil and other materials that have been contaminated with the droppings of birds that are either suffering from the disease or that have recovered and remain carriers of the *Hexamita* organisms. Recovered poults may carry the infection for many weeks and the presence of recovered birds on premises, or their introduction into an otherwise clean flock, represents the principal source of future outbreaks in susceptible stock.

It is possible that the disease may also be transmitted on contaminated utensils and clothing. Flies and other insects have not been shown to transmit it and it is unlikely that other poultry such as chickens and ducks play any part in transmission. The organism has never been found in chicken droppings. It is generally believed that outbreaks of hexamitiasis on turkey farms occur due to a build-up of infection. No trouble is experienced in the first few batches of poults but, as an increasing level of environmental contamination occurs, subsequent batches become heavily infected and eventually the typical disease results. It has also been suggested that resistant forms of *Hexamita meleagridis* occur and that these may give rise to outbreaks without any preceding build-up of infection.

Signs and Course of Disease

Signs of hexamitiasis resemble those found in many other infectious diseases. In the early stages of the **severe form**, affected poults will be noted to require more artificial heat than usual. They appear rather nervous and excitable and tend to make a continuous chirping noise. As the disease progresses they become listless and droopy, their feathers ruffled and their gait rather stilted. Appetite is diminished but water intake is normal or increased. The droppings become watery, frothy and evil-smelling. In the final stages, the poults have a thoroughly dejected and miserable appearance. They huddle together, motionless, silent and neither eating nor drinking. Soon they become comatose, fall to the ground, make a few involuntary muscular movements; death follows rapidly.

The mortality rate from the severe form of hexamitiasis can be very high. In young poults between three and five weeks of age it may approach 100 per cent. Death may occur as early as one day after signs of illness are apparent. The greatest number of deaths occur seven to ten days after onset. Mortality then slowly decreases over a three-week period and then the outbreak may terminate. In its severe form, the disease is highly contagious and may spread throughout a batch of poults within two days of the onset of signs. Recovered birds are stunted and thin, they remain underweight for several weeks and up to half of them may continue to harbour *Hexamita* organisms in the gut. These carriers of infection are a constant source of danger to healthy uninfected poults.

The **mild form** of hexamitiasis usually occurs in older turkeys of between eight and twelve weeks of age. In these outbreaks only a small proportion of affected birds show signs of ill health, and of these only a small percentage will die. Main signs shown are listlessness, ruffling of feathers, diarrhoea and some loss of appetite and condition. Poults that recover from this form of the disease may also remain carriers.

Post Mortem Findings

Post mortem findings include a thin and wasted carcase with dry, dark coloured flesh. The upper intestine is often distended with fluid and the walls are flabby, the inner lining sometimes being reddened and inflamed. The caeca, or blind guts, which are severely diseased in blackhead are not affected in hexamitiasis.

Diagnosis

Diagnosis of hexamitiasis is confirmed by laboratory demonstration of large numbers of *Hexamita meleagridis* in fluid from the upper small intestine. The organism is very small and difficult to identify under the microscope, but the fact that it is actively motile aids the diagnostician. The organisms cease to move in material taken from birds that have been dead for more than a few minutes, and so it is essential that *live* sick birds be submitted for diagnostic purposes.

PREVENTION AND CONTROL

The main control measures implemented are those which tend to reduce the numbers of *Hexamita meleagridis* in the environment of susceptible poults. Infected pens should be isolated and quarantined and be looked after by separate attendants. There should be **no communication between infected and healthy pens.** At frequent intervals, dead birds should be removed and buried or burned, the pens cleaned and the litter burned. Special care should be taken to prevent the food and drinking water becoming contaminated with droppings. Recovered birds should be isolated as strictly as possible until they are marketed.

A number of drugs have been used with varying success in the treatment of hexamitiasis but severely ill poults are unlikely to recover whatever treatment is used. **Tetracyclines** at very high levels are of some value. **Furazolidone** has also been found to be efficacious and is probably the drug of choice. Useful adjuncts to drug treatment include raising the brooder temperature and the addition of whey to the drinking water.

From the point of view of prevention, only day-old poults should be brought onto clean premises, thus avoiding the possibility of introducing carriers of the disease. All adult stock should be regarded as potentially dangerous and there should be separate attendants for the two age groups.

It is worth mentioning that the incidence of hexamitiasis has greatly fallen since the introduction of the drug **dimetridazole** for prevention of blackhead. This may be coincidence, or it may be that the drug also has some preventive effect on hexamitiasis. Little work appears to have been done to elucidate this possible additional beneficial effect of this drug.

CHAPTER 28

Worms

Worms are common parasites of poultry particularly where birds are kept on free range or on deep litter. Most species of worms do not cause dramatic clinical disease but economic loss due to depressed growth, poor egg production and lowered vitality may be considerable in heavily parasitised flocks. Only the more common worm types will be described in this chapter.

TYPES

Worms are of two main types — **roundworms** and **tapeworms** — which are readily distinguished by their characteristic shapes, the body of the round worm being round and smooth and that of the tapeworm flat and segmented. The two types also differ from each other in their method of spread from bird to bird. Roundworms produce eggs which are laid by the female into the bird's intestine; the eggs are passed in the droppings and undergo a maturation process lasting a week or more, after which they may be picked up by another bird, hatch in its intestine and there develop to a mature worm. Tapeworms also produce eggs which may be passed free in the droppings or be retained within the rear segments of the worm which periodically break off and are also passed in the droppings. These eggs, either free or within the worm segments, must then be eaten by creatures such as beetles, snails, etc.. Hatching of the eggs then takes place in the intestines of these creatures and a stage known as a **cysticercoid** develops within the body of the inter-mediate host. Only if this host containing the cysticercoid is eaten by another bird will the infestation be transmitted: eating of free eggs or segments without development of the cysticercoid will not

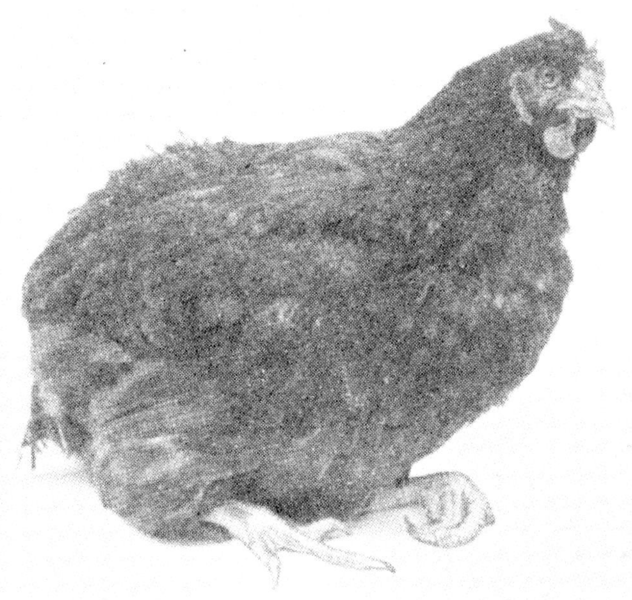

28.1   A bird heavily infested with worms. Lighter infestations are less obvious, but can have serious economic consequences.

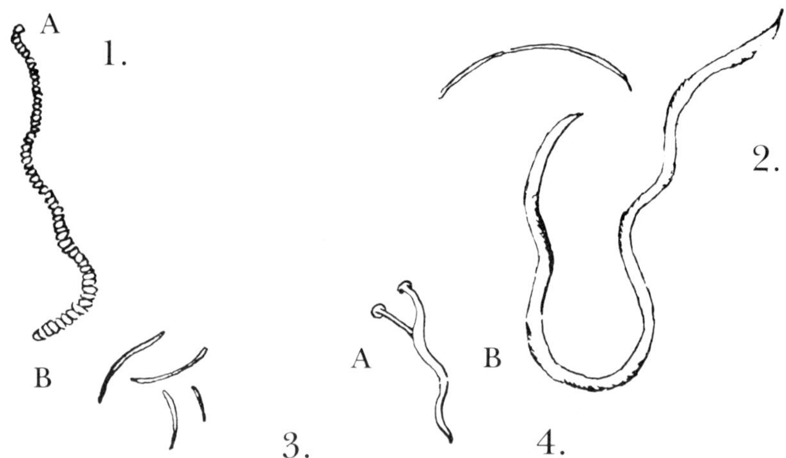

28.2   Natural size sketches of worms:
  1. Tapeworm: A.Head B.Tail
  2. Roundworm
  3. Caecal worm
  4. Gapeworm: A.Female B.Male.

result in the eggs developing into worms. Under modern conditions, birds are unlikely to have access to such intermediate hosts and tapeworm infestation has now become rare in this country. It will not be considered further except to mention that it is not uncommon in waterfowl, and is very common in certain wild game birds such as grouse, apparently having little ill effect on the host.

Roundworms

The important round worms that infest poultry include:
1. **Large roundworm,** *Ascardia galli*, which inhabits the small intestine;
2. **Caecal worm,** *Heterakis gallinae;*
3. **Hairworm,** *Capillaria*, which is also found in the intestine and occasionally in the crop; important although less common;
4. The **Gizzard worm,** *Amidostomum anseris*, a serious parasite of geese;
5. **Gapeworm,** *Syngamus trachea*, although rarely seen in poulit is a common and very troublesome parasite of young pheasants.

Large Roundworms

Heavy infestation with intestinal roundworms will result in suppression of growth rates, lowered egg production and general debility. Lower infestations probably give rise to little trouble but it should be remembered that, under certain conditions, a light infestation may build up to a heavy burden and result in ill-health.

Hairworms

Although hairworms are much less common than large roundworms, when they do occur, numbers apparently build up rapidly, and the debilitating effect on affected birds can be considerable. If untreated, many birds may eventually die.

Caecal worm

The caecal worm does not itself have much ill effect but it is of importance in that its egg acts as a carrier of the organism which causes blackhead in turkeys.

Gizzard Worm

The goose gizzard worm is a rather common parasite of young geese in which it causes severe disease of the gizzard, loss of condition and eventual death.

Gapeworms

Gapeworms are common parasites of pheasant poults and occasionally of adult birds. They are particularly frequent in wet weather conditions and in years when damp Autumn weather prevails, many pheasants may be lost. The parasites inhabit the trachea or windpipe and cause difficulty in breathing, gasping and gaping; in heavily infested birds death occurs from asphyxiation.

Signs

Signs of intestinal worms are non-specific:

1. **Large roundworms** cause loss of condition and general unthriftiness.
2. **Capillaria (hairworm)** may cause diarrhoea with inflammation of the vent and staining or loss of vent feathers and, in heavy infestations, severe loss of condition and some mortality.
3. **The goose gizzard worm** also causes loss of condition, emaciation, severe weakness and eventual death.

Post Mortem changes

Post mortem examination of birds with worm infestation in most cases readily confirms the diagnosis:

1. **Large roundworms** are easily found on opening the small intestine.
2. **Hairworms**, due to their very small size, are revealed only by a careful examination of bowel content; microscopic examination of gut content for these worms or their eggs is often helpful.
3. **The caecal worm** is also small and careful examination of caecal content is needed to show it.
4. **The gizzard worm** is easily demonstrated by its erosion of the wall of the gizzard.
5. **Gapeworms** are confirmed when opening the trachea reveals these red worms, which always occur in pairs, attached to the tracheal mucosa, together with mucus and nodules in the tracheal wall.

Treatment

Treatment by drugs is effective in most cases of infestation:

1. **Large roundworms** are effectively eradicated by giving **piperazine** compounds in the drinking water or food for one

day and repeating this in about two weeks to eliminate worms which have matured in the meantime, immature forms not being susceptible to treatment.

2. **Hairworms** are less easily dealt with, but treatment with **levamisole** is generally effective against these and **caecal worms**.

3. **The gizzard worm** was formerly treated with **carbon tetrachloride** injected into the crop but this was not totally effective and **levamisole** is probably also more effective for this parasite.

4. **Gapeworms** presented a problem for many years but **thiabendazole** in the food gave a fair measure of control. Recently new drugs have come on the market for treatment of this parasite: *Gapex* administered in the drinking water has proved highly effective, as has *Mebenvet* given in the food.

Prevention

Prevention of worm infestation depends on reducing numbers of eggs ingested by birds. Chicks should be placed on fresh litter and care should be taken to avoid introducing worm eggs on boots, etc. Worm eggs are more likely to survive on earth floors which are difficult to disinfect properly, and it is important that chicken houses be provided with concrete floors wherever possible. Worms seldom occur in caged birds because birds have little access to eggs in droppings.

Gapeworm in pheasants

Gapeworm in pheasants is difficult to prevent because of the impossibility of destroying eggs in yards or fields and the fact that eggs may be eaten by earthworms in which larvae hatch and survive for extended periods; the disease is thus transmitted to other pheasants if they eat these earthworms, which in this case act as a transport host rather than a true intermediate host.

CHAPTER 29

External Parasites of Poultry

SIGNIFICANCE

A number of parasitic species infest poultry houses and live either in cracks and crevices of the buildings, visiting birds periodically to feed (such as red mites), or in some cases spending their entire lives on the bird (such as lice). Although external parasites comprise several species of mites, lice, fleas and, in other countries, ticks, only a small number of these are widespread and of economic importance in Britain; only these important types are described below. Heavy infestations result in irritation, restlessness and ill-health with loss of production in laying flocks. Indeed, where production is rather less than expected and no other reason is obvious, the possibility of a parasitic infestation should be kept in mind.

LICE

Several types of poultry lice exist but only the **body louse,** *Menacanthus stramineus* is now commonly met in Britain. Other types comprise the head louse, fluff louse, wing louse and shaft louse. Lice are of two types, biting and sucking, but all **poultry lice are of the biting variety,** feeding mainly on skin scales and body and feather debris. The life cycle is spent entirely on the bird and lice do not survive long if removed from their host. Eggs are laid in clusters attached to the feathers close to the body and both the lice, which move rapidly among the feathers, and their eggs are visible to the naked eye. The body louse is about 3 millimetres in length and a yellow-brown colour. It is the most pathogenic louse occur-

178

ring in poultry and causes a good deal of irritation particularly of the vent region where the parasites tend to congregate in large numbers. Eventually abrasions and scabs appear round the vent and in untreated flocks the plumage becomes unkempt, flock health suffers and egg production falls.

Treatment

Treatment of lice involves application of an insecticide directly to the bird. As the parasites do not survive long away from their hosts, treatment of the building is not as important as in the case of other parasites such as red mite. A number of effective preparations are available including **gamma benzene hexachloride, pyrethrum** and **malathion** which may be applied as dusting powders or as sprays. In recent years organophosphorus compounds including **dichlorvos** and **fenchlorphos** which are highly effective and of low toxicity have become available. These are sprayed on the birds as well as the buildings and are non-toxic at correct dilution, although eggs and feed should be removed before spraying commences. A second application in about two weeks time will destroy any parasites which have hatched from eggs in the interval.

FLEAS

Fleas are seen on poultry only rarely in comparison with lice and only one species of poultry flea occurs in Britain. This is *Ceratophyllus gallinae* which is also common on wild birds and is occasionally seen on pigeons.

The poultry flea is a wingless parasite which moves by jumping. It is about 3 millimetres in length and a brownish-black colour. It can be distinguished from lice by its jumping movements and by the fact that it is flattened from side to side. Unlike lice, fleas spend much of their lives off their host. Eggs are laid on or off the bird; those which are laid on the bird being shaken off into the litter or earth where they hatch after two to sixteen days. The maggots which emerge live on organic matter in the litter until they have completed their growth, when they spin a small cocoon and pupate inside it. This may take from ten days up to a year depending on environmental conditions. Eventually the adult flea emerges to complete the life cycle.

Fleas feed on their hosts by sucking blood but frequently leave the host after feeding and can survive for many months without another meal. They cause some irritation and often congregate in

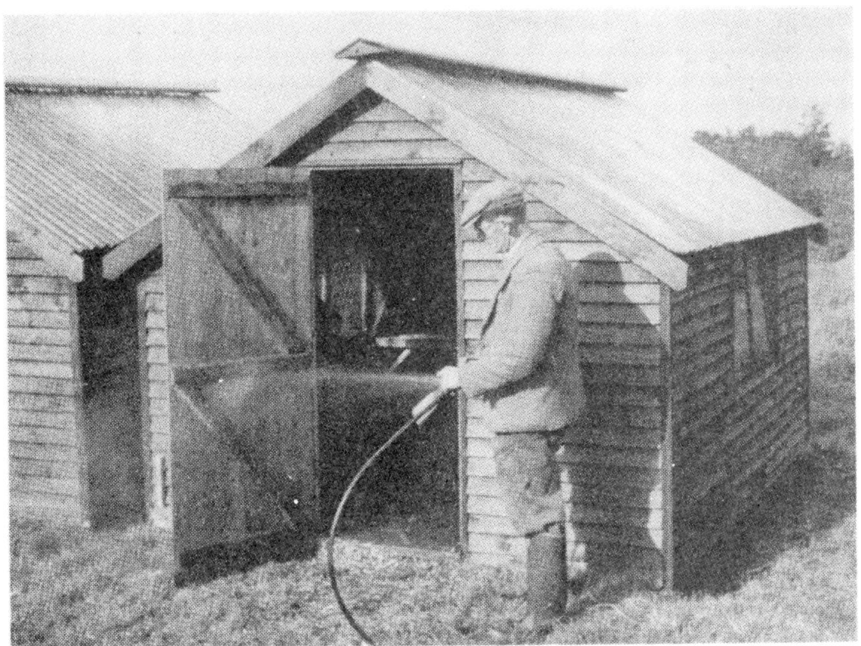

29.1   To eliminate fleas, houses should be sprayed with a suitable preparation before cleaning, and a final spraying given after the litter has been removed and burnt.

nest boxes in deep litter houses, which can lead to floor-laying by the birds. However, they are generally less pathogenic than lice and are unlikely to be a problem in caged layers.

Treatment is similar to that for lice but it is essential to **treat the house as well as the birds. Gamma benzene hexachloride** may be used to treat the birds, and the litter may have **malathion** dust added to it or both birds and litter may be sprayed with an **organophosphorus compound**. In severe infestations the litter should be removed and burned.

MITES

Four types of mites may be seen in poultry in Britain but only the red mite *Dermanyssus gallinae* is now common. It is, in fact, the commonest external parasite of poultry. The other mites, which are becoming rare in this country, are the **Northern mite,** the **depluming mite** and the **scaly leg mite.**

Red Mite

These mites are named from the red colour they assume after sucking the blood of their host. At other times they are a greyish-white colour and are easily visible to the unaided eye being rather less than 1 millimetre in length. They do not live on their host but are found in cracks and crevices in poultry houses particularly where wood is used as a construction material. They invade the host mainly at night to suck blood and then return to their places of refuge. Eggs are laid in dark cracks and corners and the mites hatch out in a few days, soon to commence blood sucking.

In severe infestations in laying houses, black spots of mite excrement may be seen on eggs. A careful search of such houses will reveal red mite in cracks and corners particularly on woodwork. Red mite can be transmitted to man and other animals causing some irritation but blood is taken only from poultry.

Red mites cause a great deal of irritation in parasitised birds. In heavy infestations birds become anaemic and a low-level mortality is possible. Egg production falls considerably and growth rates of young birds may adversely be affected. Treatment of red mite is similar to that for lice but it is most important that the **house be treated as well as the birds.** The **organophosphorus** compounds applied by spraying are suitable for this although older treatments such as **benzene hexachloride** are still sometimes used. Thorough cleaning of a house before spraying will aid the action of the insecticide. It is important when using insecticides in poultry houses to follow carefully the manufacturers' instructions with reference to dilution rate, application to birds, removal of feed or eggs and protection of personnel.

Northern Fowl Mite

This mite resembles red mite except that its entire life cycle is spent on the host. It is found mainly around the vent usually accompanied by black specks of excrement.

Treatment is similar to that for red mite but should be directed at the bird rather than the building.

Depluming Mite

This round-bodied mite attacks the feather shafts in the rump, neck and head regions causing the feathers to fall out leaving bare patches in these regions. Some disturbance in the flock results and affected birds have an unkempt appearance. This mite is rarely seen under modern conditions.

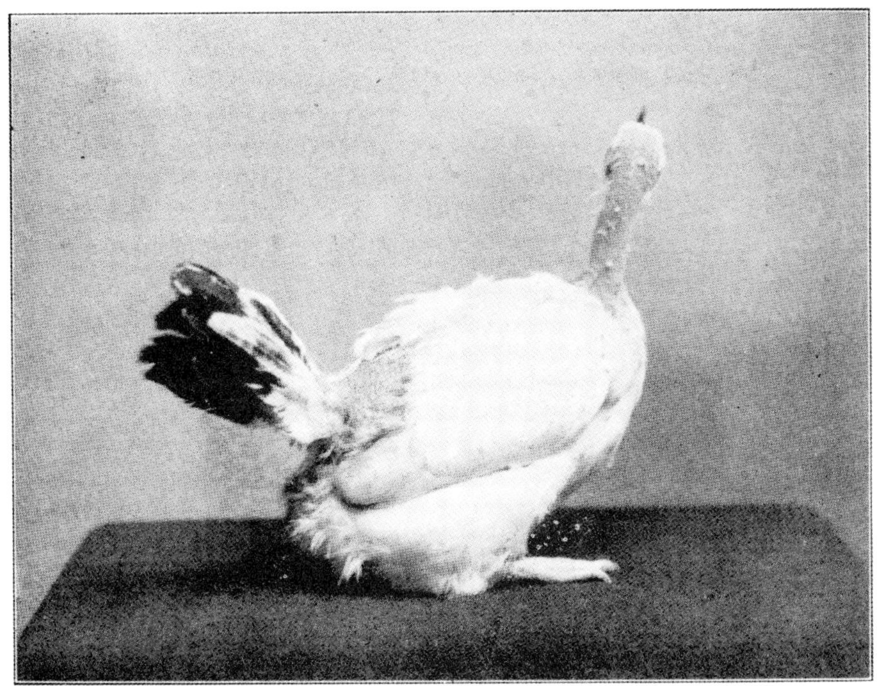

29.2   Depluming mite: note the bareness of the neck, and the part above the tail.

Treatment is similar to that for red mite but again being directed at the bird. Complete eradication of the parasite is difficult.

Scaly Leg Mite

This mite is similar to depluming mite except that it parasitises the unfeathered parts of the legs. Scaly leg is a common condition when birds are kept in small flocks on range, but is rarely seen in the modern poultry industry.

Scaly leg mites are spherical parasites of about $\frac{1}{2}$ millimetre in diameter. They burrow into the skin beneath the scales of the legs forming tunnels in which the young are produced. The scales are raised and distorted, and crusty masses of debris adhere to the legs. Irritation and lameness results and affected birds lose condition. Egg production may be seriously affected.

Treatment of scaly leg involves physical removal of loose scales and debris followed by application of a **gamma benzene hexachloride emulsion** which should be well rubbed into the affected areas. Repeated treatments may be necessary to effect a cure.

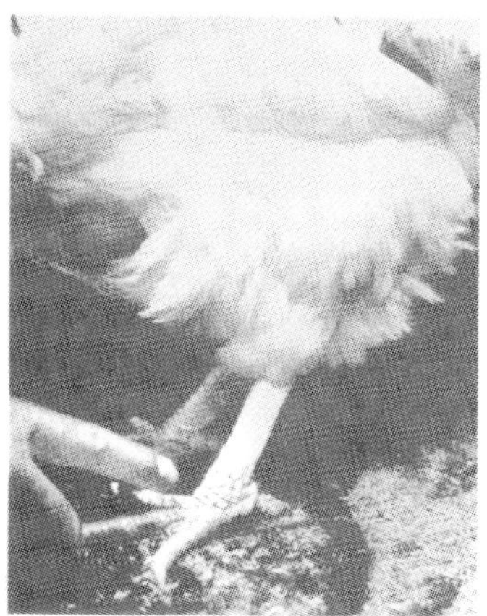

29.3 Scaly leg: note the raised scales, on the bird's legs and feet, giving a coarse, rough appearance.

In addition to the parasites described it should be said that many broiler houses are infested by various beetles, particularly *Alphitobius diaperinus;* although not true parasites, they may cause some irritation in the birds. These pests inhabit litter and walls of the buildings, and should be eradicated by spraying or fumigation of buildings between crops of birds.

CHAPTER 30

Nutritional Deficiency Diseases

In the last two or three decades, great advances have been made in the field of animal nutrition generally and, in particular, in the knowledge of precise nutritional requirements of poultry. Indeed, the scientific study of poultry nutrition has probably overtaken that of any other species. Diets for various classes of stock are now formulated with great accuracy to give maximum economic performance in the broiler and turkey growing, and egg production industries. As might be expected, accurate knowledge of nutritional requirements of poultry has led to a reduction in the number of cases of nutritional deficiency which are now encountered by poultry disease diagnosticians. Nevertheless, occasional cases of deficiency still occur and may be more dramatic than formerly because modern intensive conditions create dependence on one source of food and the bird is unable to supplement its diet by natural foraging. Signs of a deficiency in one or two birds in a flock does not necessarily indicate that the food is deficient. In the case of a gross deficiency, the signs would be widespread and other flocks on the same feed would be affected. However, whether or not disease signs are shown will depend on the degree of deficiency of the constituent concerned and the length of time for which the deficient feed is offered. Other factors such as intercurrent disease, insufficient feeder space or overcrowding may contribute to a deficiency state.

Significance of feed deficiency
In the majority of cases of feed deficiency, the deficient factors are one or more of the vitamins or minerals. These vital dietary constituents are involved in many biochemical processes within the

body so that many disease states can result from deficiencies, depending on the particular constituent which is lacking. In addition, a deficiency of protein or of specific amino acids — the building blocks from which proteins are made — may result in certain disease states or simply in poor growth, low egg production or small egg size. It should also be mentioned that deficiencies or imbalances may exert an indirect effect by making affected birds more susceptible to various infectious diseases. Some infections would be resisted by properly nourished birds in good health but may cause serious losses in inadequately fed flocks.

Difficulty in identifying deficiency

While a complete lack of one essential constituent of a ration may give rise to disease signs or post mortem changes which are specific for that particular substance, a marginal deficiency state may be more serious in the long term as the signs may be less specific and the condition may go on for a long time unrecognized. Sometimes a partial deficiency may involve more than one element of a diet, making the clinical picture even more complex. It may be some time before the diet is suspected in these cases (although farmers are prone to blame food for many problems, often on flimsy evidence!) and confirmation of a deficiency may be no easy task.

Analysis of foodstuff

Generally when a food problem is suspected, chemical analysis of the food will be necessary as an investigative procedure. In most cases the food compounder will undertake this analysis and will have the results confirmed by an independent laboratory. It is advisable, therefore, for the poultry farmer to contact his compounder when a deficiency state is suspected by his veterinarian or adviser, and to ensure that a sample of the suspect food is retained. It may well be asked, in view of the fact that the dietary requirements of poultry are now well known, why it is that flocks suffering from diseases due to faulty nutrition are still encountered: human error undoubtedly plays some part in their continued appearance. Some constituents may inadvertently be omitted during the mixing process, or included at an incorrect level. Several essential substances are perishable, or their potency can be affected by adverse environmental conditions of storage, or faulty mixing; dampness or overheating will hasten deterioration. These and other factors can upset the perfect balance at which the compounder aims in compiling the ration.

Some of the nutritional diseases to which poultry are subject are discussed below. They are disorders that have been intensively studied and which produce characteristic signs of ill-health, with consequent loss of production and still occur occasionally under ordinary farm conditions.

However most poultry rations are now formulated to contain amounts of vitamins and other microingredients more than sufficient to make up for possible losses during processing, transportation or storage so that deficiency diseases are now much less common than in earlier years.

VITAMIN A DEFICIENCY

Nature and Incidence

Vitamin A deficiency, (Nutritional Roup) common when feeding of poultry was less precise than at present, is rarely seen now. This may be due not only to more precision in ration formulation but also to the length of time that deficiency signs require to develop, much longer than the time for which a single suspect batch of feed is likely to be fed. In addition, vitamin A supplements are now stabilised to prevent loss of potency during storage. This is done either by adding anti-oxidants to the food, which prevent destructive oxidation of the vitamin, or by mechanically covering the particles of the vitamin with a layer of gelatin, wax or stable fat to prevent contact with oxygen. Adult birds, including turkeys, subjected to total deprivation of the vitamin, may not show signs of deficiency before two to five months but chicks and poults may withstand only six or eight weeks. Day-old chicks or poults receiving an A-deficient diet, and which are derived from parents whose diet was also deficient, may show signs of ill-health before they are a week old.

Signs

In young chicks and poults, signs of Vitamin A deficiency include slow growth, ruffled and broken feathers, weakness, eventual emaciation and, occasionally, signs of inco-ordination resembling avian encephalomyelitis. Yellow pigment in the beaks and leg shanks fades and the combs and wattles become pale and shrunken. The eyes may discharge a watery fluid which becomes thick and viscid, but many chicks die before this develops. Mortality can be extremely high.

Adult birds affected by vitamin A deficiency lose condition, their appearance becomes unkempt and egg production falls. Signs closely resemble those seen in respiratory disease and it is possible that vitamin A deficiency could be confused with primary respiratory infections. Breathing becomes rapid and difficult and a watery discharge from the eyes and nostrils is a prominent feature. The eyelids may become stuck together with caseous material accumulating under the lids and eventually the eyes may be totally destroyed.

In breeding flocks, hatchability is much reduced and there is an increase in the number of malpositions of the embryo.

Post Mortem Findings

Vitamin A is necessary for maintenance of healthy mucous membranes and a deficiency results in changes in the mucous surfaces of the mouth and respiratory tract. The most characteristic post mortem finding is the presence of a mass of white pustules along the roof of the mouth, extending into the oesophagus and in some cases as far as the crop. These pustules are the result of blockage of the outlets of the mucous glands due to keratinisation, or thickening, of the epithelial layer so that the glands become distended with secretions and necrotic debris. A caseous exudate may adhere to the mucous surfaces in places and the underlying surface may be dry and discoloured or ulcerated. Caseous material is often present in the facial sinuses and in the larynx and trachea. Secondary bacterial infection of these lesions frequently occurs, increasing the severity of the condition.

In some cases of vitamin A deficiency the kidneys are pale and swollen and the kidney tubules and ureters are filled with white urate deposits. These urates may also be deposited as fine film over the heart, liver and other organs giving rise to a typical "visceral gout" appearance. The clinical signs and post mortem changes of vitamin A deficiency may not be sufficiently characteristic to differentiate the condition from various respiratory diseases and fowl pox. This can only be done by histological examination of affected tissues and in cases of doubt it will be necessary to submit live affected birds to a laboratory equipped to undertake this work. It must be said however that vitamin A deficiency would be regarded as a rare disease under modern conditions of management and feeding. It is unlikely that a grossly deficient ration would be formulated and fed for a period sufficiently long to produce signs of deficiency. Respiratory infections on the other hand are still

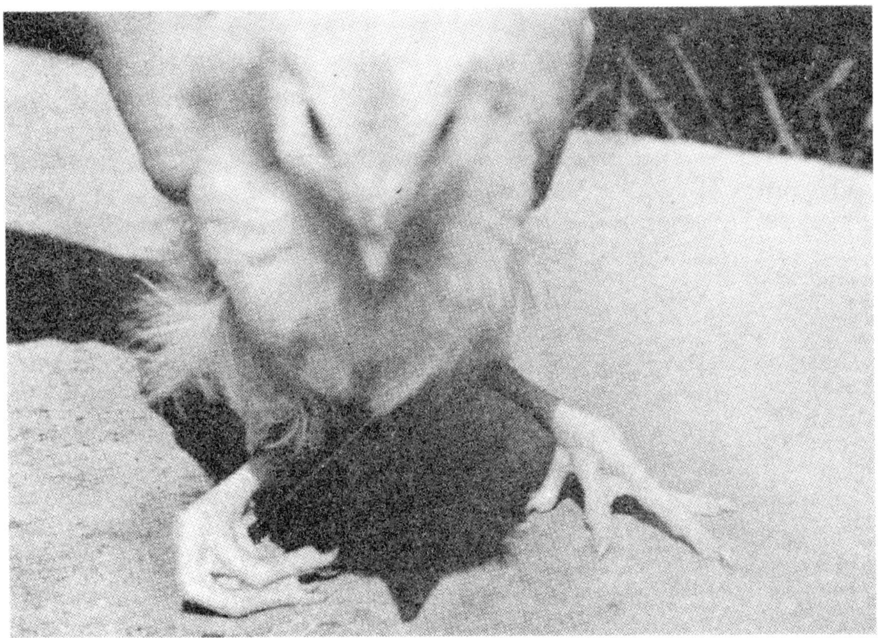

30.1 Riboflavin deficiency (curly toe disease) in a chick.

relatively common. The latter therefore are a much more likely cause of respiratory signs than the former, and in any investigation of disease in which these signs are present, vitamin A deficiency would be considered a possibility only if other more common diseases were considered and eliminated.

Treatment

Chickens and turkeys respond rapidly to the addition of vitamin A to the ration. The vitamin is best given as a stabilised preparation at a level of 3000 to 5000 I.U. per pound of feed for a period of two to three weeks. Most birds recover on this treatment and egg production is restored relatively quickly.

Cod liver oil may be used as a source of vitamin A, but since this material may reduce the availability of vitamin E it should be used with caution.

VITAMIN B COMPLEX

Nature and Incidence

The vitamin B complex includes a number of essential substances the chief of which are thiamine (B.1), riboflavin (B.2), nicotinic acid, pantothenic acid, pyridoxine, biotin, folic acid, choline and cyanocobalamin (B.12).

It is often difficult to differentiate the individual vitamin B members from one another according to the signs they produce in deficient birds. Young, growing birds are generally affected more than adults. In general the principal signs include loss of appetite, retardation or cessation of growth, poor feathering, nervous signs and leg problems. Deficiencies of some members of the group, for example thiamine, are almost non-existent under practical conditions and they will not be considered further. A brief description follows of deficiency signs of some which may be seen from time to time although it should be emphasised that none is met with commonly under modern conditions.

Riboflavin

This is generally added to the feed as a supplement since the main dietary ingredients of most rations contain insufficient amounts.

Signs

Deficiency signs occur in both young chicks and unhatched embryos derived from flocks fed on deficient diets. In embryos, the main manifestation of the condition is an abnormality of the down in which the developing feathers are retained within their sheaths so that the feathers appear as beads or knots instead of the normal feather shape. The abnormal feathers are most common on the neck and breast and the condition is referred to as "**clubbed down**".

Clubbed down may also be seen in newly hatched chicks, but in growing chicks up to three weeks of age which are fed deficient starter diets the most characteristic sign is an inward and forward curling of the toes generally referred to as "**curled toe paralysis**". Birds suffering from this condition have difficulty in walking and maintaining balance and tend to sit on their hocks. A rather similar condition used to occur when chicks were brooded under infra-red lamps but in this condition the toes curled sideways and the birds were less disabled, generally walking on their feet rather than sitting on their hocks.

It should not be assumed, when a few chicks in a flock are found showing curled toes, that the whole flock is necessarily suffering from riboflavin deficiency. If this is the case many birds will show paralysis without curled toes and if the sciatic nerves, the main nerve trunk to the legs, are examined, they will be found to be thickened and yellowish in colour.

Treatment
In riboflavin deficiency severely affected chicks should be culled, but if the deficiency is corrected the flock will generally make a rapid recovery.

Folic acid and Choline

Deficiency of these substances is uncommon under practical conditions, but they play a part in prevention of perosis (slipped tendon) and a deficient diet may precipitate cases of perosis particularly where there is a tendency for these to occur due to other causative factors.

Signs
Other signs of deficiency include anaemia, poor feather growth and pigmentation, and a paralysis of the neck in turkey poults.

Treatment
Deficiency signs can be rapidly corrected by addition of high levels of folic acid to the diet.

Biotin

This member of the B complex has come into prominence in recent years due to its involvement in fatty liver and kidney syndrome. (This is considered in a separate chapter.) In addition to this disease, however, it is well known that biotin deficiency gives rise to a separate syndrome in which skin lesions are prominent. It has not yet been fully explained why these two conditions, both apparently due to biotin deficiency rarely occur together in the same flock, although it should be added that the skin lesions are much more commonly seen in turkey poults than in chickens and that turkeys do not appear to suffer from fatty liver and kidney syndrome.

Causative Factors
The cereal base of the diet appears to affect the development of deficiency signs. Wheat based diets are frequently low in biotin and supplementation of such diets is necessary to ensure adequate biotin intake in poults to which they are fed. In some cases the

biotin content of a diet is theoretically adequate but its availability to the bird is reduced due to its being present in the intestine in a bound form. Some biotin is synthesised by intestinal bacteria but the extent to which this can be utilised by the bird is uncertain.

Signs

Signs of biotin deficiency include slow growth, poor feed conversion, leg problems including slipped tendon and skin lesions. These consist of thickening of the skin of the undersides of the feet with eventual cracking, fissuring and haemorrhage. Scab formation at the corners of the beak and around the eyes may also occur. Biotin deficiency should be suspected when these signs occur, but confirmation of deficiency by laboratory estimation of levels in feed is difficult and results may not be easily interpretable.

Treatment

Treatment of biotin deficiency is by addition of the vitamin to the feed or drinking water. Skin lesions heal relatively quickly when adequate levels are made available to the birds but leg deformities, although they may be improved, will not be completely resolved.

VITAMIN D DEFICIENCY

Nature and Incidence

Although vitamin deficiency diseases are rather uncommon now, a deficiency of vitamin D in starter or grower rations, resulting in rickets, probably occurs more frequently than most deficiency diseases. A similar condition occurs in the case of a severe calcium deficiency, phosphorus deficiency, or a large imbalance in the relative quantities of calcium and phosphorus in the ration. In most cases, however, rickets is due to lack of vitamin D in the diet. Destruction of the vitamin in the finished food is slow and cases of deficiency are probably due more often to mixing errors then to in-feed deterioration.

Vitamin D prevents rickets by promoting the absorption of calcium from the intestine. Without Vitamin D, absorption of calcium is inefficient, resulting in inadequate mineralisation of bone and development of a typical case of rickets. Blood levels of calcium are maintained by a hormone secreted by the parathyroid glands and, in cases of rickets, an increase in the size of these minute glands, which lie at the entrance to the chest, can be detected.

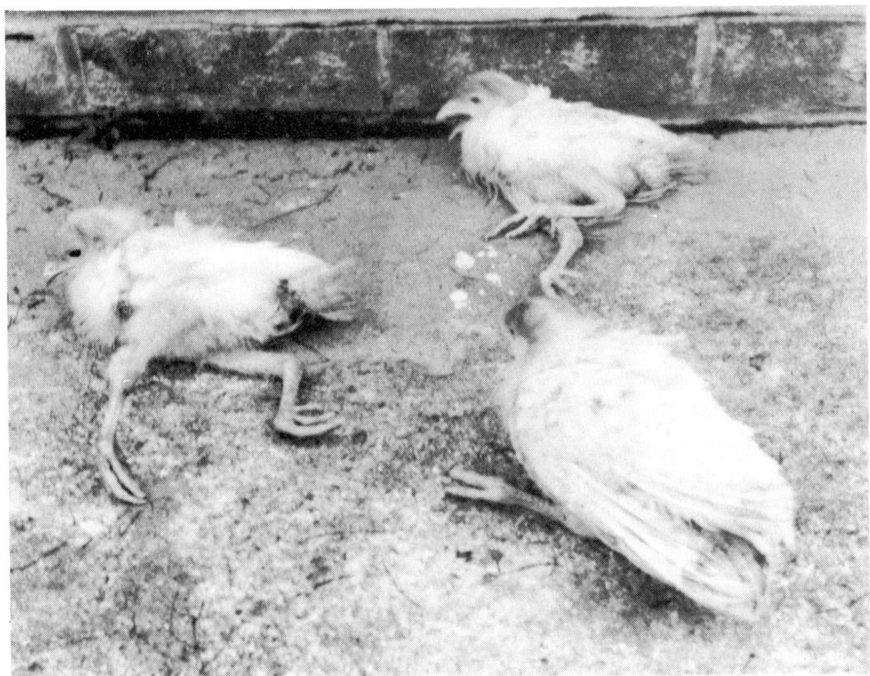

30.2 Rickets in turkey poults. When poults of two to six weeks go off their legs, Vitamin D. deficiency rickets should be suspected.

Vitamin D Deficiency in chicks

Signs

In most cases of rickets, signs first become visible at two to three weeks of age, although this depends on the age at which a deficient ration is fed. Chicks or poults lack vigour, grow slowly and have poor feathering. Frequently however, the first sign noted is leg weakness; chicks are unwilling to move and, if forced to do so, take only a few unsteady steps before squatting down again or sitting back on their hocks. Other causes of leg problems may give rise to similar signs and post mortem examination is necessary to confirm the diagnosis.

Post Mortem Findings

In a typical case of rickets, the most obvious finding is a soft condition of the long bones, which tend to bend, rather than break with a definite snap, as occurs in the normal chick. The beak is also flexible, and the ribs may be distorted and show swellings at their junctions with the vertebral column.

There may be visible swelling and distortion at the growing ends of long bones particularly the femur and tibia, but this feature is not usually as obvious as in mammalian rickets.

The part played by the parathyroid glands in rickets has already been mentioned. These are difficult to see in the normal chick but may be enlarged to pea-size in the rachitic chick.

Diagnosis

Rickets should be suspected when chicks or poults of about two to three weeks of age suddenly show leg weakness with softness of bones. An increase in thickness of the growth plates of long bones and typical changes in the ribs and parathryoid glands will add to the evidence.

Analysis of a feed sample to establish the levels of vitamin D^3 (the most active form of the vitamin for poultry), calcium and phosphorus is essential for confirmation of the diagnosis. It should be noted that estimation of levels of vitamin D^3 is difficult, expensive and time consuming. Vitamin A levels, however, are easily estimated, and are often used instead of D, on the assumption that since both vitamins are added to the feed together, the level of one reflects the level of the other.

Histological examination of the growing ends of long bones, in which disturbed growth and mineralisation will be apparent to the pathologist, is also sometimes used as additional confirmatory evidence of rickets.

Cases of rickets not infrequently occur in which feed levels of calcium, phosphorus and vitamin D and their ratio to one another are normal. These cases have been called "field rickets" and their cause is still unknown.

Treatment

When rickets is confirmed the poultry food should be replaced by food containing correct levels of vitamin D, calcium and phosphorus. In most cases the flock will make a relatively rapid return to normal. Vitamin D can be supplied in concentrated form to individual birds in cod liver oil, if this is considered necessary.

Vitamin D Deficiency in Adult Birds

In adult birds, deficiency of vitamin D or calcium gives rise to thinning and weakening of long bones, and softening of the beak, nails and keel bone. Egg production falls and many soft shelled and shell-less eggs are produced. These changes occur relatively slowly, taking up to three months to appear, depending on the degree of deficiency. Some birds in cages show a temporary paralysis of the legs which has been called **cage layer fatigue**. Death may follow quickly but many recover if taken out of their cages and hand-fed. This condition is not invariably associated with a deficient diet, but is in some cases apparently due to an inability on the part of the bird to reduce egg production when bone calcium has been grossly depleted. The bones are brittle and fractures may occur, but egg shells are normal and on post mortem examination an egg is often present in the oviduct.

Treatment of laying birds

Treatment of calcium or vitamin D deficiency in laying birds depends on ensuring adequate levels are present in food. In many cases a rapid response is obtained by sprinkling limestone or oystershell grit on the food. The same procedure in high producing flocks once or twice a week may prevent production and shell problems or an outbreak of cage layer fatigue.

VITAMIN E DEFICIENCY

Nature and Incidence

Vitamin E is another compound which is essential to the continued health of poultry flocks. This vitamin is involved in the normal functioning of many tissues of the animal body and a deficiency of it may give rise to a number of syndromes in a variety of animal species. In the chick or poult three distinct conditions may result. These are:

1. **Nutritional encephalomalacia or "crazy chick disease"**
2. **Exudative diathesis**
3. **Muscular dystrophy.**

All occur in young birds. Adults show no signs of deficiency, although hatchability of eggs from vitamin E deficient flocks may be reduced due to death of embryos at about three days of incubation.

Chemically, vitamin E is a mixture of compounds known as **tocopherols** which occur in green food generally and particularly in maize and wheat germ oils. The most active form is **d-**

alpha-tocopherol. The action of these compounds is complex but they are believed to prevent destruction of other essential chemical compounds within the body. They are readily destroyed in feeds which are going rancid, particularly in the presence of oils such as cod liver oil. Vitamin E however can be partially replaced in diets by other chemicals such as **ethoxyquin** which have anti-oxidant properties. In addition, the element **selenium** has some of the disease-preventing properties of vitamin E although it is not related to it chemically. An apparent vitamin E deficiency therefore may not indicate a straightforward deficiency of the vitamin but may be related to the degree of rancidity of the food, the level of anti-oxidants and selenium and the content of substances such as cod liver oil, as well as the actual level of the vitamin present. Because of these complicating factors, care should be exercised in interpreting the significance of vitamin E levels in diets.

Nutritional Encephalomalacia

As already mentioned, vitamin E deficiency may give rise to three syndromes, separately or in combination. The best known of these syndromes in Britain is nutritional encephalomalacia or crazy chick disease. In this condition, which affects chicks or poults up to four or five weeks of age, nervous symptoms predominate.

Signs

Movement is unco-ordinated, the chicks lose their balance and stagger drunkenly or fall over backwards. Uncontrolled movements of the head and neck may occur or the neck may twist round in a circular fashion so that the bird looks up at the ceiling. Finally paralysis occurs, the bird is unable to get to its feet and death soon follows. Mortality levels of 5 to 10 per cent may be expected but the sooner a diagnosis can be made and the chicks given supplementary vitamin E the lower mortality will be.

Post mortem findings and diagnosis

There are no visible pathological changes in the internal organs in crazy chick disease. Only in the brain can changes be seen, characterised by oedematous swelling and haemorrhages scattered over the surface of the brain. In many cases, however, histological examination of the brain is required to differentiate the condition from others such as epidemic tremor in which similar signs may be evident; for this purpose live chicks should be delivered to a suitably equipped laboratory. Distinctive changes in the brain are usually clearly visible to the pathologist. Vitamin E levels in feed may be estimated but this is a difficult and expensive procedure and, as already mentioned, difficulties may arise in interpretation of the results.

Treatment

Removal of feed and its substitution by fresh feed containing adequate vitamin E and anti-oxidants should be carried out as soon as the diagnosis is confirmed. Addition of a vitamin mix including vitamin E to the drinking water may also be beneficial. **Severely affected chicks will not recover** and should be destroyed.

Exudative Diathesis and Muscular Dystrophy

These conditions frequently occur together although they are not often seen in Britain. They apparently occur where selenium levels in the ration are low as well as those of vitamin E and they can be prevented by ensuring adequate selenium levels in the food.

Signs

In **exudative diathesis** there is accumulation of clear or greenish fluid under the skin of the breast region and wings as a result of increased permeability of capillaries. There may also be fluid within the pericardial sac and haemorrhages are usually present in the breast muscle.

In **muscular dystrophy**, white streaks are visible in the breast and thigh muscles indicating areas of muscular degeneration. Ducklings are apparently more susceptible to this type of lesion than chickens. In turkey poults the muscle of the gizzard is frequently affected.

Treatment

Treatment of these conditions is by addition of correct levels of vitamin E and selenium to the diet. In the case of muscular dystrophy the levels of cysteine and methionine should be checked and corrected if necessary. Synthetic anti-oxidants have no effect.

MINERAL DEFICIENCIES

In addition to the vitamin deficiencies just described, deficiencies of minerals also occur. These elements are equally essential to the health and well being of poultry and a number of well defined syndromes are recognised as being due to deficiency states. The most important minerals which may on occasion be lacking in feeds are **calcium and phosphorus, salt (sodium chloride), manganese and zinc.** Experimental deficiency of various others e.g. potassium, iodine, iron and copper can be produced but seldom occur under practical conditions.

A short description of deficiencies of the more important minerals follows.

Calcium & Phosphorus Deficiency

These elements are required for normal bone formation in the young chick and for egg-shell formation in the laying bird. A deficiency of either, or an imbalance of the two, in a ration will give rise to a state of rickets in young chicks. There are differences in the precise alterations to developing bones which occur depending on whether the cause is calcium or phosphorus deficiency or their imbalance, but generally the signs shown are the same; lameness and softening of bones. It should be noted that the majority of cases of rickets are due not to actual shortage of these elements but to a deficiency of vitamin D which results in reduced absorption of calcium from the intestine. (Rickets has been discussed under vitamin D deficiency.)

In adult birds lack of calcium and phosphorus gives rise to shell-less and soft shelled eggs and brittleness of bones. This has also been discussed.

Salt Deficiency

Salt is essential for many life processes and lack of it in chicks or poults will lead to reduced appetite, poor growth, dehydration and high mortality. In the laying bird egg production falls, food consumption decreases and severe feather pecking and cannibalism may occur.

Although salt deficiency in food is not unknown, excess salt with its attendant syndrome of excess drinking and loose droppings is probably more common.

Manganese Deficiency

Deficiency of manganese in poultry rations has been recognised for many years as the cause of the condition known as **perosis or slipped tendon.** Manganese is normally added to poultry food as a supplement, the quantities in natural ingredients being insufficient for health and optimal growth. Absorption from the intestine is reduced by high levels of calcium and phosphorus in the food.

Perosis symptoms

Perosis occurs in young growing chicks or poults. The hock joints become enlarged and distorted and the lower end of the tibia frequently becomes bent or bowed resulting in slipping of the Achilles (or gastrocnemius) tendon from its normal position on the rear of the hock. Affected birds become severely lame and if both legs are involved, may die due to inability to reach food and water.

It should not be assumed that every case of slipped tendon is due to manganese deficiency. Indeed under modern conditions the cause of slipped tendon may be complex, with genetic influences, deficiencies of other substances such as choline and biotin and other conditions such as twisted leg, which result in distortion of the hock joint, all having a possible causative effect. Determination of the precise cause can, on occasion, be difficult and time consuming.

Treatment

In cases where manganese deficiency is shown to be the cause, the food should be substituted by a ration containing adequate quantities of manganese. This will prevent further cases developing, but correction of advanced cases of leg deformity and slipped tendon will not occur.

In laying birds manganese deficiency results in lowered egg production and hatchability, with severe physical deformity of embryos, many of which die in the later stages of incubation. Egg shell quality is also affected.

CHAPTER 31

Lameness & Leg Conditions

One of the commonest causes of loss to the modern poultry industry is the occurrence of various types of lameness and leg weakness in the growing bird, both broiler and turkey. The causes of some of these conditions are known, but in other cases, in spite of much investigation and research the causes have not been fully established.

The modern table bird is bred and fed for maximum growth rate in the shortest possible time and this already remarkable performance level is still being increased by the geneticists and nutritionists. There is little doubt that an increased incidence of leg abnormalities is an undesired effect of these accelerating growth rates; it would appear that skeletal strength has barely kept pace with body growth and that this is the underlying cause of a number of leg abnormalities and lamenesses. It has been convenient to describe some leg conditions such as staphylococcal arthritis, manganese deficiency and rickets in other chapters of this book. It should be borne in mind that lameness and paralysis may result from nervous, muscular and infectious causes as well as from actual skeletal conditions. Some additional important conditions will be discussed in this chapter.

VIRAL ARTHRITIS

Viral arthritis or tenosynovitis is an infectious disease of chickens, mainly of meat-type birds, caused by a *reovirus*. It occurs in many countries including Britain although its incidence is not high in this country at present.

Spread

The means of transmission of the disease is uncertain but egg transmission probably occurs, followed by rapid lateral spread between birds in a flock by direct contact. Infection of flocks with the virus may be much more common than clinical disease would suggest and it is believed that maternal immunity may play some part in resistance to the virus.

Signs

The disease is most common in broilers of five to six weeks of age and upwards. Most infected birds show no signs but where clinical evidence of disease is present, signs include lameness, poor growth and swelling of the tendons and tendon sheaths in the region of the hock joints and shanks. Mortality is not usually high although losses of up to 16 per cent have been reported.

Post Mortem Changes

Post mortem findings include swelling of tendons in the hock and shank areas and some blood tinged fluid in the hock joint. There may be haemorrhages in the synovial or lining membranes of the joints, and erosions in the joint surfaces in chronic cases. It is believed that infection of the tendons with the viral arthritis agent predisposes to **rupture of the Achilles tendon** (described below).

Diagnosis of viral arthritis can in many cases be made with some accuracy from the appearance of the lesions considered in conjunction with the anti-mortem signs. Sometimes, however, it may be impossible to distinguish between this disease and others such as staphylococcal arthritis or infectious synovitis, and confirmation of diagnosis depends on isolation of the virus from affected tissues.

Treatment

There is no treatment for viral arthritis. Antibiotics have no effect on the virus. **Affected birds should be culled** and the usual hygiene and disinfection measures taken to prevent spread of infection to other flocks.

TIBIAL DYSCHONDROPLASIA

This is a condition of the knee joint of broiler chickens, ducks and other table poultry which is seen from about five weeks of age onwards. It has been recognised for a number of years and has been studied by a number of prominent workers, but it is still incompletely understood.

Signs

The condition has become rather common in broiler flocks although many affected birds show no lameness or other clinical signs. Only in severe cases are signs like swelling of the knee, lameness and reluctance to walk likely to be seen.

Post Mortem Changes

Advanced cases are readily diagnosed at post mortem examination by the swelling in the knee joint region, bowing of the tibia and the characteristic plug of uncalcified cartilage which is seen beneath the growth region at the upper end of the tibia, on longitudinal splitting of the bone. In severe cases, the upper end of the tibia is bent backwards due to weakness of the bone at this point, sometimes resulting in fracture at the point of bending. Occasionally cartilage plugs are also found at the upper end of the metatarsal bones. The condition is unlikely to be confused with any other, although less severe cases may bear a superficial resemblance to rickets.

Cause

The cause of tibial dyschondroplasia is still uncertain but no infectious agent is involved. The condition has a hereditary basis but it will become manifest only if certain environmental or nutritional factors happen to be present. The fast growth rate of the modern table bird is believed to be involved in this as in so many other leg problems, and it has been shown that a high chloride level in the food will predispose to the condition. If chloride, in salt for example, is replaced by bicarbonate, the incidence of the condition is reduced. The actual cause is believed to be an interruption in the blood supply to the upper tibial growth plate although how this is brought about is uncertain.

Treatment

There is no treatment for tibial dyschondroplasia. The condition does not respond to addition of minerals or vitamins to the diet. Although the condition is not at present of great significance to the broiler industry it could become so if geneticists and nutritionists continue to produce heavier and faster growing birds without at the same time giving consideration to skeletal strength. Even at

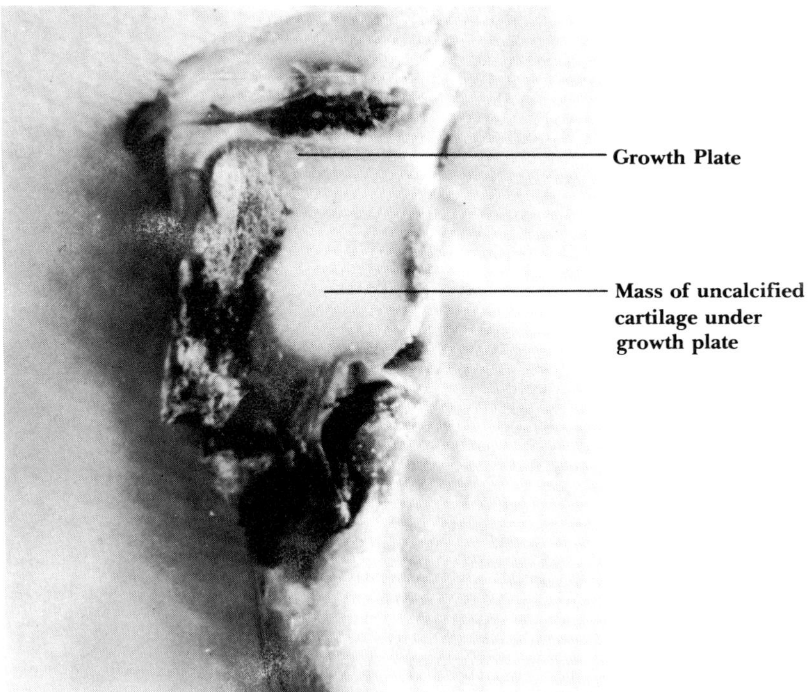

31.1 Tibial dyschondroplasia. Upper end of tibia (leg bone) split lengthwise to show uncalcified cartilage 'plug' below the growth region.

present, although few birds in a flock may show signs of the disease, some may be downgraded or require to be trimmed in the processing plant due to abnormal conformation of the legs.

TWISTED LEG

This is a common condition in broiler flocks, although in most cases only a small number of birds in a flock are affected. It is also seen in turkeys and occasionally in pheasants.

Signs
It is characterised by a deformity of the hock joint, usually of one leg only, in which the bones immediately above and below the joint are bent and twisted resulting in various, and often bizarre, angulations of the affected leg. In some cases the gastrocnemius tendon slips from the point of the hock, but the term perosis should not be used to refer to this disease.

Cause

The cause of twisted leg is uncertain but it is probably due in part to damage to the lower tibial growth plate during hatching or at a later stage, resulting in deformity of the joint.

Treatment

No treatment is available for the disease; affected birds grow poorly and **should be culled.** If they are allowed to survive to killing age, downgrading or trimming of the carcase in the processing plant will be inevitable.

SPONDYLOLISTHESIS

This condition of broiler chickens is popularly known as **Kinky Back** and results in apparent lameness or birds going off their legs. Unlike most other conditions described in this chapter, it is not due to an abnormality of the legs, but rather to a paralysis resulting from damage to the spinal cord.

Signs

The condition is common in broiler flocks but, as in the case of twisted leg, usually only a small number of birds are visibly affected. Most cases appear after the age of four weeks. Affected birds tend to adopt a rather characteristic attitude of squatting on the rump with both legs pushed out in front. They are unable to get on their feet, and attempts to do so often result in the bird progressing backwards.

Cause

The actual cause of spondylolisthesis is a deformity of the spinal column at the level of the sixth thoracic vertebra. It is thought that immaturity of the chicken skeleton combined with the very rapid growth rate of the modern broiler, causes the vertebral column to become deformed at this point, with resulting compression of the spinal cord and paralysis of the legs. The condition apparently develops within the first two weeks of life and it has been shown that it can be prevented by restricting food intake and growth rate at this early stage of the bird's life. There is also a hereditary predisposition.

Diagnosis

The condition is quite easily diagnosed from the ante-mortem

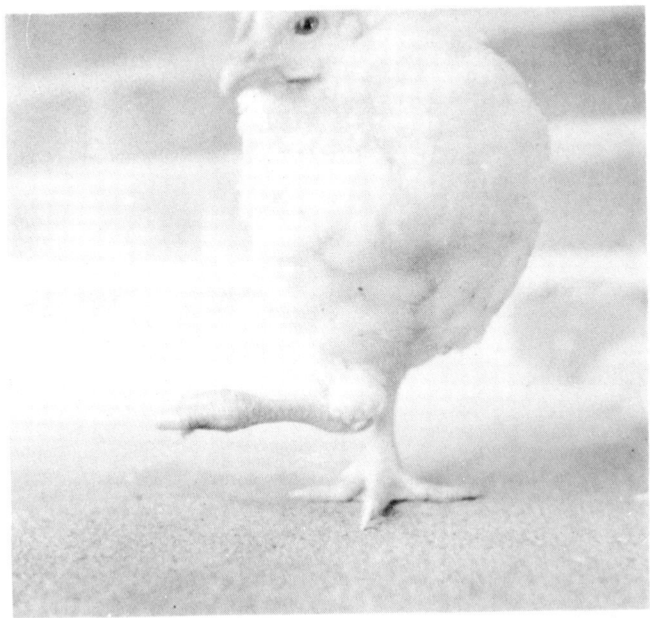

31.2   Distortion and angulation at the hock joint. A form of twisted leg.

signs and demonstration at post mortem examination of displacement of thoracic vertebrae with spinal cord compression. Longitudinal splitting of the spinal column usually shows this lesion clearly.

Treatment
There is no treatment for affected birds which **should be culled**. If they are allowed to survive they will grow poorly due to inability to reach food and water and may eventually die of starvation.

RUPTURED GASTROCNEMIUS TENDON

This condition, known popularly as **Green Legs,** is occasionally seen in broiler flocks, usually in a small number of birds, but is much more common in broiler type birds which are grown on to a killing age of twelve or fourteen weeks following caponisation. It is likely that the extra weight of these large birds contributes to the condition by placing additional strain on the tendons. In this disease there is probably also a hereditary predisposition. In capon flocks, up to 5 per cent of birds may be affected and one or both legs may be involved. Although the disease is not directly due to an infectious agent, it has been found that some cases of viral arthritis are followed by ruptured tendons and there appears to be an association between the two conditions.

Signs

Rupture of the gastrocnemius tendon, which attaches to the back of the hock, takes place just above the hock and is accompanied by haemorrhage in this region. The lesion shows externally as a blue-green discoloration of the skin surrounding the point of rupture. In bilateral cases affected birds are off their legs, unable to stand upright and they "walk" on their hocks. When only one leg is affected, the bird shows a pronounced lameness of that leg. Incision through the skin of a recent case shows swelling, haemorrhage, accumulation of inflammatory fluid; the rupture of the tendon is easily visible. In long-standing cases healing of the ruptured ends of the tendon takes place and firm nodular swellings may be felt under the skin. Affected legs are unmarketable, resulting in considerable economic loss if significant numbers of birds are affected.

Treatment

No treatment is available; affected birds are best culled and the flock should be killed and marketed as soon as possible.

SHAKY LEG SYNDROME

This is an abnormality of the legs of growing turkeys, usually seen in birds of eight to twelve weeks of age or older.

Signs

It is a form of leg weakness in which the main feature is a shaking or quivering of the legs when affected birds rise to their feet after a period in the sitting or resting position. There is apparently some difficulty in rising, an unwillingness to walk and a resumption of the sitting position after a few steps. Some affected birds can be found in the majority of turkey flocks, but recently an increased incidence of the condition has been reported. The cause is unknown but is apparently associated with a weakness of the neck of the femur or thigh bone.

Concomitant factors

The significance of this syndrome is uncertain; some birds or flocks apparently recover, but in others the condition becomes progressive and bird performance suffers. Frequently there are associated abnormalities of structure and posture, such as bowing of the legs, a "rolling" gait and a hunched and tipped forward posture.

Treatment

There is no treatment for shaky leg syndrome nor any known means of prevention. Further work is required to establish the precise nature and cause of this interesting condition.

SPRADDLE LEGS

This is an abnormality of the legs of young chicks in which the legs splay out sidewards or in front. It appears to be due to hatching difficulties or to chicks being placed on a slippery surface soon after hatching. It is important that both the hatching trays and the material on which baby chicks are placed should be non-slippery so that they gain a firm footing.

Chicks affected by spraddle legs should be culled.

CROOKED TOES

In this condition, which may be seen in birds of any species, the toes are turned either medially or laterally. They are not, however, turned under the foot as in curled toe paralysis of riboflavin deficiency, and lameness, difficulty in walking, or similar symptoms are not features of the condition. The cause is unknown but a similar condition used to occur when chicks were brooded under infra-red lamps and excess exposure to infra-red rays was said to be responsible. Cases still occur although infra-red brooding is seldom used nowadays and it is likely that other causative factors including heredity are of significance. As the condition apparently causes no inconvenience to affected birds it is of little clinical or economic importance except for exhibition birds.

PLANTAR PODODERMATITIS

In this condition, there is **necrosis** and **ulceration** of the underside of the foot with resulting pain and lameness in some cases, although some birds in which the condition is present do not appear to suffer any ill-effects.

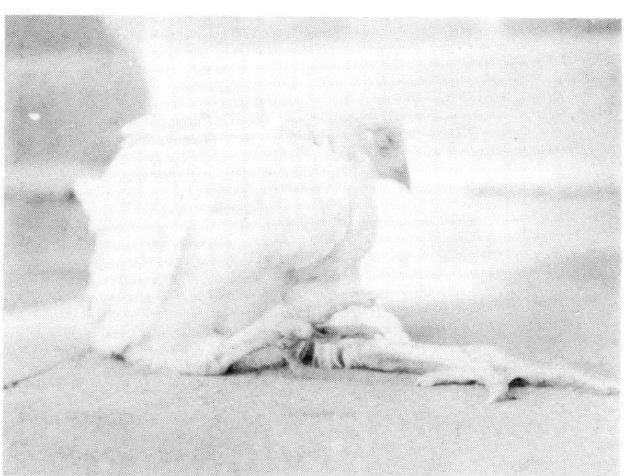

31.3 Spondylolisthesis (kinky-back): six week old broiler showing typical posture. Bird sits on rmp supported by hocks.

The cause is apparently related to improperly managed litter which has been allowed to become excessively wet or has solidified. It has been suggested that some types of diet will give rise to accumulation of irritant substances in the litter with resulting foot problems. The condition is also occasionally seen in semi-free range birds, kept on an insufficient area of ground which becomes churned to little better than a mud bath in periods of wet weather.

ARTICULAR GOUT

This condition, occasionally seen in older birds, is a result of accumulation of urates in leg and toe joints. These urates, normally excreted in the urine are deposited in joints and other situations (visceral gout) due to kidney malfunction. The joints become swollen and painful, and incision into an affected joint will show a white, chalky urate deposit. The condition is probably more common in budgerigars and other cage birds than in hens.

CHAPTER 32

Miscellaneous Diseases

In addition to those diseases which occur in outbreak form, affecting many birds in a flock and sometimes many flocks in an area, there are a great many conditions which occur sporadically, affecting only a small number of birds and are generally of only minor significance. Most are non-infectious, some are associated with management and the causes of some are unknown. These conditions, however, form an interesting group which should not be overlooked. Some, for example **degenerative myopathy in turkeys**, are the subject of research projects.

A brief description of the more important of these conditions is given in this chapter.

DISEASES OF THE REPRODUCTIVE TRACT

Since poultry have been specially bred for high egg production, it is not surprising that the reproductive tract is subject to malfunction and disease.

Egg peritonitis and internal laying

Although non-infectious, these conditions are often seen in laying birds in association with infectious diseases such as Newcastle Disease. They commonly occur also in birds approaching peak production when a secondary *E.Coli* infection is often superimposed. The cause is the failure of yolks released from the ovary to enter the oviduct so that they drop into the abdominal cavity. Here they accumulate, with the result that the abdomen becomes filled with a solid or semi-solid mass of yolk material. Affected birds stop laying and most eventually die either from the condition itself, or from secondary *E.coli* or other infection. In some cases, the yolk material spreads out as a solid mass engulfing most of the abdominal organs. Egg peritonitis is easily diagnosed at post mortem.

Treatment

There is no treatment for uncomplicated egg peritonitis but where *E.coli* infection is involved and significant mortality is occurring, appropriate antibiotic treatment may give some beneficial effect. Little can be done by way of prevention, other than avoidance of rough handling, sudden fright or other stress factors.

Conditions of the oviduct

Impaction of the oviduct occurs when the oviduct, the tube down which the egg passes before laying, becomes obstructed with egg material. This may be caused by disease or stricture of the oviduct or by an abnormally large or malformed egg. As more material accumulates the oviduct may rupture and an egg peritonitis condition result. Oviduct impaction and egg peritonitis often occur together.

Eversion or prolapse of the oviduct refers to a condition in which the oviduct is pushed out through the vent. This may result from a number of causes including incorrect feeding of pullets, which come into lay with too much body fat, and incorrect lighting programmes that bring immature pullets into lay too early before the oviduct muscles and vent tissues are properly developed. Another causative factor may be too sudden increase in day-length resulting in ovulation defects, particularly production of double-yolked eggs.

Prolapse of the oviduct generally results in death of the affected bird and in addition a prolapse problem may precipitate a cannibalism outbreak with loss of a significant number of birds.

No treatment, other than the possibility of surgical correction in a valuable breeding bird, is of any value for this condition. Prevention depends largely on correct rearing procedure, avoiding over-fatness, correct lighting patterns and debeaking of the flock at an appropriate stage during rearing.

DISEASES OF THE DIGESTIVE SYSTEM

Alimentary Impaction

Probably the commonest non-infectious condition affecting the intestinal tract is **impaction or obstruction**. This used to be rela-

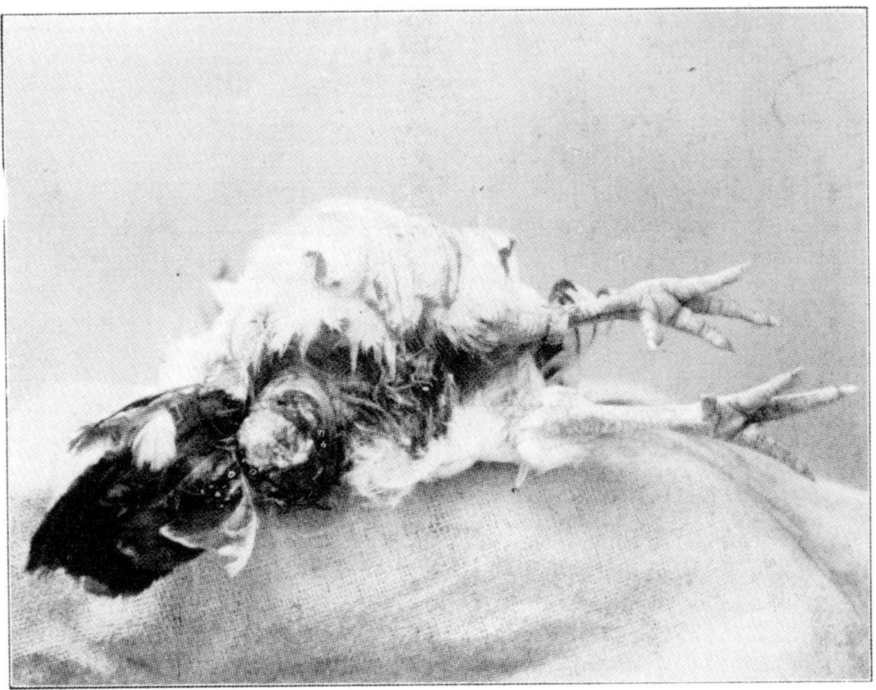

32.1   Prolapsus of the oviduct, in this case, the portion of the oviduct protruding contained an egg.

tively common when birds were kept on free range and was due to eating coarse grass or similar fibrous material. It is now rare in laying birds but still occurs not infrequently in turkey poults where chopped straw is used as litter. Poults often begin to eat straw, a habit which rapidly spreads until quite a significant number of birds are lost. Since straw may also give rise to aspergillosis in turkeys, use of this material for turkey litter is inadvisable except in emergency. Sometimes even the more commonly used wood shavings give rise to a similar condition. Impaction usually occurs in the gizzard with the impacting material often extending into and dilating the duodenal loop. Occasionally the mass escapes from this site only to obstruct a lower part of the small intestine.

The condition is easily diagnosed at post mortem, the offending mass being found in the gizzard or intestine. No treatment is of any value. Prevention depends on not allowing birds access to material which may be eaten and give rise to the condition or, in serious cases, removing the material where losses are already occurring.

Provision of a suitably sized insoluble grit may have some beneficial effect.

VENT PASTING

This is a condition of young chicks in which a mass of dried faecal material adheres to the feathers around the vent. The vent is blocked and the terminal part of the bowel is distended by accumulated faeces which the chick is unable to pass. The condition is usually due to some irritation of the bowel which causes passage of fluid faeces. This may be a specific infection of the bowel or due to early stress factors, poor quality feed, etc.. It sometimes accompanies yolk sac infection.

Antibiotic treatment may be beneficial where bowel infection is involved. Physical removal of the obstruction may cure individual cases.

PENDULOUS CROP

This condition was at one time fairly common in turkeys and is also occasionally seen in adult hens in which it is usually referred to as **sour crop.** In turkeys there was believed to be an inherited predisposition. Increased water intake in hot weather may also be a causative factor but in many cases the fungal infection Moniliasis, or thrush, is involved.

The crop becomes loose, enlarged and baggy. It seldom returns to normal size, never empties properly and remains filled with a sour liquid. The lining may ulcerate and bacterial infection supervene. Many affected birds die although some survive for long periods in an unhealthy condition. Treatment of pendulous crop is not advisable. **Affected birds should be culled.**

Volvulus

Volvulus, or twist of the bowel, is not uncommon as a cause of isolated losses in various ages of birds. The bowel becomes twisted upon itself, its blood supply is interrupted and the affected part becomes distended and of a dark purplish colour. Affected birds die rapidly from severe shock. Losses are sporadic; the condition should not be confused with coccidiosis.

Vent Gleet

This condition, an inflammation of the vent with a characteristic and offensive odour, was rather common some years ago but is

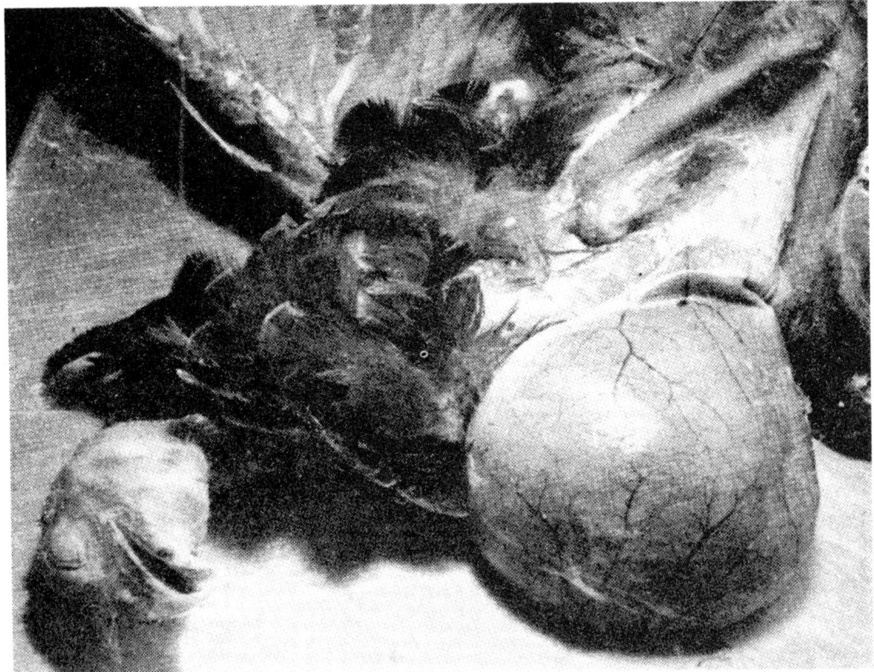

32.2 Pendulous crop in a turkey. The part is not impacted but seriously distended owing to a weakness of the crop wall.

rarely seen now. The cause is unknown; there is some doubt as to whether it is infectious.

There is a white discharge from the vent with matting or loss of vent feathers. The tissues around the vent become reddened and swollen, and ulceration may occur. Affected birds may show discomfort and straining and their egg production is much reduced.

Treatment is not generally considered worthwhile, affected birds being culled. However, in the case of valuable birds, cleaning up the vent area followed by repeated applications of a mild antiseptic solution or antibiotic ointment may effect a cure.

URINARY TRACT CONDITIONS

The kidneys are affected in a number of diseases of birds including Mareks disease, infectious bursal disease and nephrotoxic infectious bronchitis, known in Australia as Cummings disease. Surveys have shown that "nephrosis/nephritis" conditions (disease of the kidneys) are commonly involved in mortality in laying flocks.

The causes of these latter conditions however, are not specified and there is a need for further work to investigate the significance of kidney disease in birds.

Visceral gout

Visceral gout is a result of kidney malfunction rather than a disease of the kidneys themselves. It is a rather common condition of mature birds and occasionally occurs also in young chicks in which it is sometimes referred to as **baby chick nephrosis.**

The cause in some cases is undetermined; in others it is associated with infectious disease, especially nephrotoxic infectious bronchitis. It is well known and often quoted that a high protein diet will predispose to the condition but it is doubtful if this is a frequent cause under practical conditions. Shortage of water is also sometimes suggested as a cause and deficiency of Vitamin A may on occasion give rise to the condition. In baby chicks, the cause has not been determined although "stress factors" are sometimes quoted as a rather non-specific cause. A high calcium diet will damage the kidneys of young chicks and in cases of visceral gout in baby chicks it should be ensured that the food contains the correct level of calcium.

Signs

Signs of Visceral gout, which usually affects only a small proportion of a flock, are depression with loss of appetite, shrunken comb and loss of condition; death occurs in a few days.

Visceral gout is due to malfunction of the kidneys with the result that urates, which are normally excreted in the urine, accumulate as a white chalky deposit on the surface of the liver, pericardium, other internal organs and the subcutaneous tissues. The kidneys are enlarged and urate deposits are also visible in the kidney tubules and in the ureters, which may be distended to several times their normal thickness. The condition is easily diagnosed at post mortem from the characteristic chalky urate deposits. These changes are distinct from the post mortem picture in coli septicaemia and the two conditions should not be confused.

Treatment of visceral gout will depend on determining the cause and treating or correcting this if possible. In some cases a number of birds are lost from visceral gout over a short period, the cause is undetermined and the problem stops as suddenly as it started. In any case of visceral gout it should be ensured that adequate supplies of water are available to all birds in the flock.

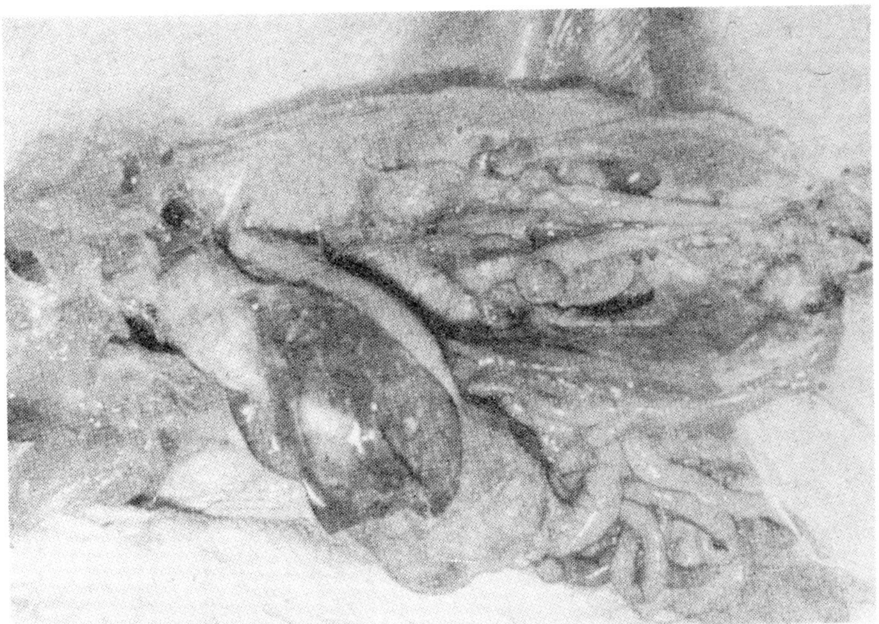

32.3   A case of visceral gout. The heart and kidneys are covered with white deposits of urates, and the ureters are distended with this material.

FATTY LIVER HAEMORRHAGIC SYNDROME

Fatty liver haemorrhagic syndrome is a disease of poultry, peculiar to egg layers, which is characterised by sudden death of a variable number of birds in a flock. The condition was first reported in America in 1954 and since that time has been seen in many other countries, including Britain. It is not a disease of major importance on a national scale but nevertheless can be a significant problem to the individual egg producer whose flock is affected.

Occurrence

The disease occurs in laying flocks mainly of the heavier, brown-egg laying breeds. Outbreaks are sporadic but tend to occur in caged birds in periods of warm weather.

Cause

The precise cause of the condition is not known but no infectious agent is involved and spread from bird to bird does not occur. Dietary factors are believed to be involved, chief of which is excess consumption of carbohydrate, or "energy". This carbohydrate is converted to fat in the bird's body and stored in various fat deposits, including the liver, with the result that the liver becomes enlarged, pale in colour and soft or friable. Eventually, rupture of the liver capsule or surrounding membrane occurs and the bird dies almost immediately from massive internal haemorrhage. It has been suggested that the tendency to lay down fat internally may be increased by the fact that most laying birds are now confined in cages which, by restricting movement, reduces their requirement for energy. In addition, many cage houses are now maintained at higher temperatures than formerly, which again may contribute to the problem by reducing maintenance energy requirements. If these theories are correct the disease may be said to be due to intake of energy in certain birds in excess of that which is required for maintenance and production under modern conditions of environment and housing.

It will be appreciated that the above description of cause is vastly over-simplified, the precise biochemical processes terminating in excess deposition of fat in the liver being long and complex. In addition various workers have implicated other factors among which must be mentioned the apparent increase in liver haemorrhage with increasing levels of rape seed meal in the diet and the possibility that diets deficient in lipotropic factors (chemical substances such as choline which mobilise fats deposited in the liver) may contribute to the problem. Clearly, although much progress has been made, further work is required to elucidate the complex causative influences in this condition. It should be mentioned finally that there is no connection between this disease and fatty liver and kidney syndrome in younger birds. The causes of the two conditions are entirely unrelated.

Signs

Usually there are no premonitory signs of the condition. If any fall in egg production occurs it is unlikely to be more than a few per cent. It may, however, be noticed that a significant number of birds in the flock are overweight due to excess fat deposition in the abdomen. This will be particularly evident if birds are handled. Some birds may appear nervous or flighty. Frequently, however, the flock owner notices nothing untoward until a slight increase in mortality occurs.

Post Mortem Findings

The post mortem findings in this condition are quite distinctive.

On opening a carcase the cause of death will immediately be obvious — a large blood clot lies free in the abdomen, having originated from rupture of an enlarged, yellowish, soft, mushy liver. In addition, there are large deposits of yellow fat in the abdominal cavity which may make the bird considerably overweight. In some cases, evidence of previous, smaller, non-fatal haemorrhages under the liver capsule may be found, suggesting that a tendency to massive fatal haemorrhage has existed for some time. There are generally no other significant changes although the kidneys may also be pale and swollen. Internal laying and egg peritonitis are not usually features of the disease. Frequently a normal egg is present in the oviduct of birds that have died from the condition.

Microscopic examination of the liver will reveal a heavy infiltration of fat with distension and rupture of many cells, yet this does not appear to have much effect on the general health of the bird until the final gross liver rupture occurs.

Mortality due to the condition is generally low, rarely exceeding 2 to 3 per cent. A persistent low-level mortality, however, can be a source of some concern, in addition to financial loss, to a flock owner who may suspect an infectious disease in his flock. A post mortem examination will soon allay these fears.

Treatment

Until further knowledge of the precise cause of the condition becomes available, treatment should be aimed at reducing the energy intake of the flock either by restricting feed intake or by altering the components of the diet. It is known that the amount of fat deposited in the liver following conversion from carbohydrate varies depending on the main source of carbohydrate in the diet; maize produces more fat than barley, and so, changing the cereal base from maize to barley could be beneficial. The possibility that an alteration to diet may upset egg production should be considered before such a change is made, particularly in a high producing flock suffering only minor mortality from the disease.

Prevention

The nature of the disease and its sporadic occurrence make it unlikely that any definite preventive measures will be taken before an outbreak occurs. However, a flock owner who finds that a significant number of his birds are overweight should bear the condition in mind; any preventive measures taken should be the same as those following an outbreak.

FATTY LIVER & KIDNEY SYNDROME
NATURE AND INCIDENCE

Fatty liver and kidney syndrome is a disease of young chickens of both broiler and pullet type which was first described in Denmark in 1958 and has since become common in many countries including Britain. The condition has also been called **Pink Disease** or "**Pinks**" from the discoloration of the carcase which occurs in birds dead of the disease.

The condition has given rise to considerable mortality particularly in broilers, but is now largely controlled since the discovery of the involvement of the vitamin **biotin** in the disease. Cases still occur but are generally less severe than formerly.

Cause

Although a great deal of research has gone into a study of the disease the precise cause is still uncertain. However it is known that no infectious agent is involved and spread from bird to bird does not occur. The condition is believed to be the result of a complex interaction of dietary and environmental factors. It has been shown that wheat-based diets containing low fat and protein levels tend to give rise to the condition and the energy to protein ratio is also important. How these nutritional factors cause the condition is not fully understood, but recently it has been found that an important role is played by the vitamin biotin.

The actual cause of death in fatty liver and kidney syndrome is believed to by **hypoglycaemia or low blood sugar.** Sugar is formed in the liver from certain constituents of the diet and biotin is involved in this biochemical process. When biotin is deficient, sugar formation is impaired, glycogen reserves in the liver are used up (particularly during periods of stress), blood sugar levels fall and death eventually results from low blood sugar. This is a much simplified account of the process; the precise biochemical abnormalities which lead to hypoglycaemia and fat deposition in the liver and other organs are extremely complex.

It is known that **pelleting of feed increases susceptibility** to fatty liver and kidney syndrome and this may be due to destruction of biotin by heat of pelleting. Where birds are kept on wire, access to biotin in their droppings is restricted and susceptibility to the condition is increased.

Signs

There are few visible signs associated with the disease. Often the best grown birds in a flock are affected. They become dull, appetite is lost and death soon follows. The finding of dead birds however, is often the first indication of the disease in a flock.

A number of years ago mortality due to fatty liver and kidney syndrome sometimes reached 20 per cent. Since the discovery of the role of biotin, its inclusion in rations of parents and broilers has tended to confine mortality to a few individual birds. However, flock outbreaks still occur, possibly more commonly now in pullet flocks than in broilers.

Post Mortem Findings

The flesh of birds dead of fatty liver and kidney syndrome often shows a reddish-pink discoloration. This may also be noted in the fat tissue. Rapid degeneration and disintegration or "rotting" of an affected carcase may be noted.

Internally the most obvious features are the pallor and swelling of the liver and kidneys. The liver is soft and mushy, and sometimes small haemorrhages may be noted particularly around the edges. The kidneys are also soft and swollen but urate deposits are not a feature. The changes in the liver and kidneys are due to fatty infiltration which also occurs in other organs including the heart and intestinal tract.

In many birds dead of the disease there will be found a black-brown coloured fluid in the gizzard and upper small intestine. The nature and significance of this fluid is uncertain.

Treatment

Since it is now known that the disease can be prevented by addition of biotin to the food of chicks, this addition has become routine and outbreaks requiring treatment have now become uncommon. When such an outbreak does occur, addition of biotin to the drinking water may be effective. It has long been known that treatment with **molasses in the drinking water** has some beneficial effect and this is believed to be due to its biotin content.

A method of "treatment" commonly used in days before the role of biotin in the disease was known, was a short period of starvation. This would now be considered a stress factor which could precipitate an outbreak, yet it must be said that withdrawal of food did, in some cases, appear to have a beneficial effect in that it stopped mortality: this apparent anomaly requires explanation.

Prevention

Fatty liver and kidney syndrome is now prevented by addition of biotin to the ration of chicks and their parents. This routine has become so successful that other preventive methods need scarcely be considered although avoidance of stress factors is also important. An increased protein content of the diet may help to prevent the condition.

KERATOCONJUNCTIVITIS

This condition, known as **Ammonia Blindness,** occurs due to improperly managed litter giving rise to excess ammonia fumes in the house resulting in damage to the surface of the eye. It is seen in broiler, pullet and turkey flocks, usually in young birds in winter, and although not as common now as in the earlier years of intensification of the poultry industry, still occurs occasionally where management and hygiene practices are sub-standard.

Cause

Although the prime cause is high ammonia levels from litter, poor ventilation and overcrowding are contributory causes. Affected birds appear dejected, stand with closed eyes and lose condition as they fail to eat and drink. A sign of the condition is constant rubbing of the eyes against the wing. Examination of the eye of an affected bird will show swelling of the eyelids, conjunctivitis and ulceration of the centre of the cornea, or surface of the eye, giving it a "frosted-glass" appearance.

The condition is apparently painful. Affected birds prefer to remain in dark corners and occasional characteristic cries or "squaks", due presumably to pain, may be heard in a house in which the condition is present.

Treatment and Prevention

No treatment appears to be of much value but birds will slowly recover if removed from the source of ammonia. Prevention depends on correct litter management, providing adequate ventilation to remove ammonia fumes, and avoidance of overcrowding.

A new condition

Recently, a condition apparently identical to ammonia blindness has been seen in a number of flocks; it differs in that demonstration of a significant level of ammonia in affected houses has not been possible. Flocks on litter are usually involved and it has been noticed that new cases cease to appear as soon as flocks are caged in their laying quarters. There appears to be an association with litter, as cases appear following scratching or dust-bathing in litter, but the precise cause is still unknown. Some cases have apparently responded to antibiotic treatment while in others this has had no effect. Further work is required to determine the nature of this interesting condition.

MYCOTOXICOSIS AND TURKEY X-DISEASE

Nature and Incidence

Mycotoxicosis is a type of poisoning due to contamination of food or litter with metabolites produced during growth of certain species of fungi. The best known example of this disease complex is **turkey X-disease** which caused considerable losses among growing turkeys in the early 1960's.

Mycotoxicosis

Although mycotoxicosis is not frequently diagnosed in this country, it may well be more common than generally suspected, as a cause of reduced performance rather than severe disease with mortality. Certainly in countries with hot and humid climates, conditions which favour fungal growth, mycotoxicosis can be a source of considerable loss to the broiler and egg industries.

It is important to distinguish between mycotoxicosis due to ingestion of preformed fungal toxins, and mycosis due to growth of fungal elements themselves, in or on the animal body.

Cause

Fungal elements and spores are extremely common in nature and their growth is supported by various media including ingredients of chicken feed, the finished feed itself and litter. Not all types cause disease or produce harmful toxins, but, in tropical countries in particular, mycotoxins can be detected in a large number of grain and feed samples. The main toxin producing species are *Aspergillus flavus* and *A.ochraceus*, *Fusarium* species and *Penicillium citrinum*. The toxins produced are known as Aflatoxin, Ochratoxin A & B, Trichothecene (T-2), Zearalenone (E-2) and Citrinin.

Chickens acquire the toxins by eating contaminated food or litter. Spread from bird to bird does not occur.

Signs

Signs of mycotoxicosis are varied and non-specific depending to some extent on which toxin is involved. They include reduced growth rate, poor feathering, diarrhoea, sometimes with blood, thirst, reduced egg production and mortality. Losses may vary from negligible to 20 per cent or more, depending on age of bird and toxin type and concentration.

Post Mortem Findings

These are also variable and include widespread haemorrhages particularly in muscles and in the intestinal tract, enlarged spleen and liver and pale bone marrow. Neither the signs nor the post mortem changes are specific for mycotoxicosis and diagnosis depends on identification of toxins in feed or other source. Identification of these however is a specialised laboratory procedure for which few laboratories are equipped and in some cases a presumed diagnosis from signs and post mortem changes may have to suffice.

Prevention

Prevention of mycotoxicosis depends largely on prevention of fungal growth and toxin production in feed or other material to which birds have access. Grain should be harvested at the correct time and properly dried and stored; maize with over 14 per cent moisture content should not be used in poultry feed. Storage bins in feed mills and milling equipment should be dry and moisture and humidity in the mill kept to a minimum. Any mouldy material should be removed and destroyed and an appropriate sanitation programme instituted. Treatment of feed with chemical substances (organic acids) will help to prevent fungal growth and various preparations are available commercially for this purpose.

Bulk bins on farms should be kept clean, dry and free of fungal growth. It should be ensured that the insides of bins are free from pockets of stale food. Food should not be stored for any longer than necessary and litter should be kept dry and feed spillage onto litter avoided.

It must be said that the prevalence of fungi is such that in spite of all preventive measures, cases of mycotoxicosis continue to occur. Treatment of the disease in live birds is valueless. **Removal of the**

source of toxin is the only practical method of controlling an outbreak.

Turkey "X" Disease

This was a particular type of mycotoxicosis which occurred in turkey flocks in England in the early nineteen-sixties causing the death of approximately 100,000 turkey poults. They showed signs of depression, drooped wings, ruffled feathers, loss of appetite, nervous derangement, neck spasm and death with the legs stretched out rigidly backwards. A search for the cause of the syndrome eventually showed the involvement of a toxin in a ground nut consignment purchased from Brazil. This was an **aflatoxin** produced by the fungus *Aspergillus flavus*. Several flocks of ducklings were also affected and it was shown that ducklings are more susceptible to the toxin than turkeys.

Post Mortem changes

The main pathological change occurred in the liver which was swollen, firm and pale in colour. The kidneys were congested and swollen and there was amber coloured fluid in the pericardial sac. In some cases there was generalised oedema of the carcase. Diagnosis of the disease can be confirmed by histological examination of the liver in which specific, well defined changes are seen.

Prevention

The syndrome is well known to feed compounders today and feeds are screened for the presence of aflatoxins. However it could still occur if feed is incorrectly stored after delivery to the farm. Hence the importance of correct, short-term storage so that the growth of **Aspergillus** or other moulds is prevented.

DEEP PECTORAL MYOPATHY

Nature and Incidence

This condition, first detected in America in 1967 and a little later in Britain, is an abnormality of the deep breast muscles (supracoracoid) of turkeys. Since its discovery, the condition has received a number of names including **Oregon Muscle Disease** (from the fact that much of the early work on it was done at Oregon State University), **green muscle disease, hereditary myopathy** and **degenerative myopathy.**

The condition occurs mainly in spent turkey breeder hens; it has also been recorded in broiler breeders, but is rarely if ever seen in young growing birds. The incidence in affected flocks varies from as little as 2 per cent up to 35 per cent, and various strains of bird have been affected. The importance of the condition lies in the possibility of affected carcases getting onto the market and the product image of turkeys suffering when the affected tissue is found by consumers on cooking and carving such birds.

Cause

Although a good deal of research work has been done on the condition its precise cause has not yet been determined. Various theories have been advanced including physical damage due to handling, injections of vaccines or antibiotics into the affected region, nutritional factors and unspecified environmental influences. Infectious agents have been ruled out as possible causes.

Recently it has been shown that a partial failure of, or interruption to, the blood supply of the affected muscle is partly responsible for the condition. The reason for this abnormality of blood supply is still being investigated. It is also known that hereditary factors are involved, females being more affected than males.

Signs and Post Mortem Changes

There are no detectable clinical signs and the condition poses no threat to the health or well-being of affected birds in life. Detection of the lesion is possible only at post mortem examination. Only the supra-coracoid, one of the deep muscles of the breast, is affected; the condition may be unilateral or bilateral. A slight elevation or depression may be visible without incising the breast, but incision and removal of overlying muscle is necessary to show the lesion. The appearance of the affected muscle varies depending on how long the condition has been present. The typical change is usually present in only the middle third of the muscle. In early cases there is swelling, pallor and moistness of the affected muscle but there is no green discoloration. Later the swelling and moistness subside and the area assumes a greenish colour, while in long-standing cases the green colour becomes more pronounced, the tissue becomes dry, brittle and shrunken and a thick fibrous capsule develops around the lesion and separates it from the surrounding tissue. Sometimes haemorrhages are present in the region of this capsule and the underlying bone may be eroded where the muscle lies against it. In these chronic cases the anterior third of the muscle is normal while the posterior part is often pale and atrophied or wasted.

Diagnosis

In the live bird diagnosis is not generally possible; cases come to light on the line in the slaughter plant.

The importance of preventing affected carcases reaching the market has already been mentioned and to this end a number of attempts have been made to devise a reliable means of detecting these carcases. The difficulty lies in the fact that the affected tissue is a deep muscle lying against the keel bone and completely covered by normal muscle tissue. It can only be revealed by incising and reflecting the overlying muscle. This is costly, however, and will result in many unaffected carcases being cut, thus reducing their market value. Some affected carcases can be detected by visual inspection, the affected side of the breast being either swollen in early cases or slightly contracted in chronic cases, giving the breast region an asymmetrical appearance. This inspection will not detect all cases, however, since in some carcases the alteration is too slight to be noticed and in others, which are bilaterally affected, carcase symmetry is not apparently altered. Handling of carcases to detect a depression or swelling may help in diagnosis, but this again is not sufficiently reliable.

Work in recent years at the Food Research Institute in Norwich has resulted in the development of a "light-probe", a powerful light in a tubular steel case; the tube is inserted into the carcase cavity following evisceration and the breast region examined by means of the light shining through the carcase muscle. A lesion shows up as a triangular shadow in the region of the keel bone. This method of detection has proved to be much superior to any other yet devised.

Treatment and Prevention

There is no treatment for the condition, even if cases could be diagnosed in the living bird. Hereditary factors are involved, therefore it may be possible in future to eliminate the defect by selective breeding. This, however, would depend on development of a reliable means of detecting early cases in life. Much further work will be necessary if this is to be achieved.

AORTIC RUPTURE

Nature and Incidence

This condition, **which occurs only in turkeys,** can be a cause of significant mortality and of considerable economic loss, since well grown male birds twelve weeks of age and over are usually affected. The main feature of the disease is sudden death of a number of birds in a flock, losses ranging up to 5 per cent, although 1 per cent or less is more usual. Birds are usually found dead but occasionally one may be seen to die when the flock is frightened or disturbed.

The cause of death is massive internal haemorrhage due to rupture of the aorta, the main arterial outlet from the heart; the abdominal portion is usually affected, although on rare occasions the rupture may take place in the thoracic portion. Rupture of the vessel is a consequence of a degenerative process of the internal lining. The lesion is known as **dissecting aneurysm** and although it has been the subject of a good deal of research its precise cause is still uncertain.

Cause

Dietary factors, including high protein and high fat have been implicated and high blood cholesterol levels are believed to be involved. It has also been observed that chemical caponisation is sometimes followed by a high incidence of aortic rupture. The relative importance of these various factors remains to be determined. A major factor in the actual rupture process is believed to be the remarkably high blood pressure of the turkey, which may rise sharply even higher if birds are disturbed or frightened, or during fighting in males.

Post Mortem Diagnosis

Aortic rupture is easily diagnosed at post mortem examination. Even without opening the carcase the condition may be suspected from the pallor of the wattles and flesh, resulting from internal haemorrhage. A large blood clot found in the abdomen, or occasionally in the thorax, confirms the diagnosis. Although other conditions such as **erysipelas** can cause sudden death in turkeys of the same age the conditions are readily differentiated at post mortem.

Treatment

Treatment of the condition is not possible as no premonitory signs are shown but the inclusion of a "sedative", **reserpine** in the food of susceptible birds has a preventive effect. This drug apparently lowers blood pressure in the turkey and this is probably more important than its sedative effect. Flocks in which losses have occurred should be disturbed as little as possible until they are marketed.

ROUND HEART DISEASE

Nature and Incidence

This is a condition of chickens and turkeys in which the heart becomes enlarged and distorted or mis-shapen, and which is characterised by sudden death of apparently healthy birds due to heart failure. The condition has been seen in various parts of Europe, the U.K., New Zealand and Canada, although it is rare in the U.S.A..

In the nineteen-fifties, the condition was common in Scotland and Northern England. It was seen mainly in the winter months in Leghorn and Rhode Island Reds and their crosses, usually in pullets, although it has been recorded in birds of one month to nineteen months of age. It is less common now than formerly.

Cause

The cause of round heart disease has never been determined although a number of suggestions have been put forward. When it was at its height it occurred mainly in birds on deep litter and has never been recorded in cages. Its present decreased incidence may be associated with the fact that the vast majority of layers are now kept in cages. It was believed that litter had some causative effect, particularly since it was found possible to induce it in birds placed on litter taken from premises where an outbreak had occurred. It was suggested that a toxin absorbed from litter might be involved.

Other theories as to cause have included zinc poisoning, Vitamin E or selenium deficiency and an inherited predisposition. There is no evidence that any infectious or parasitic agent is involved in round heart, and transmission experiments have been consistently unsuccessful. It may be that the cause of the condition is complex, several factors being required to operate concurrently for an outbreak to occur.

Signs

The first indication of the disease may be sudden death of birds in good condition which were apparently in good health a short time earlier. These sudden deaths may occur when birds are excited such as at feeding time, or if they are caught for examination or other reasons. Deaths are apparently due to sudden failure of a diseased heart.

Occasionally in the course of an outbreak some birds may be seen to be in poor condition, lethargic, with pale or bluish comb or wattles. Most of these birds will die although some may recover. The death rate in an affected flock may reach 50 per cent but usually it is much lower. Losses may continue in a flock for a few weeks but there is no great tendency for the condition to spread to other flocks even if they are in relatively close contact.

Post Mortem Changes

Most birds dead from round heart disease are in good bodily condition although some may be rather light. The main changes are found in the heart itself. It is enlarged, up to twice normal size and its walls are thickened. The normal cone-shape is lost, the apex becoming rounded or blunt with an indentation or 'dimple" at its peak. The colour becomes a yellowish-pink, the musculature assumes a parboiled appearance and the heart veins become swollen and engorged. In some cases the pericardial membrane surrounding the heart is distended with clear, yellow-tinged fluid.

Changes in other internal organs are due to malfunction of the diseased heart. The liver becomes swollen and dark in colour due to damming back of venous blood and some clear fluid (ascites) may be present in the abdominal cavity. A gelatinous coat may envelop the liver and the lungs may be water-logged.

Since the cause of round heart disease is unknown no specific treatment can be applied. Vitamins and trace elements have been used apparently with some beneficial effect, but antibiotics have not given any useful results. Changing the feed and water have been reported to be partially effective.

In view of the possible connection between litter and outbreaks of the disease, removal and changing of the litter during an outbreak and use of fresh litter for each flock are advisable measures. Until more becomes known about the cause of the disease further useful measures cannot be suggested.

OEDEMA SYNDROME

This is a condition of turkey poults of about four days to two weeks of age in which the main change is an accumulation of fluid in the body cavities and tissues. Affected poults show little evidence of clinical disease but are usually found dead, often lying on their backs.

Post mortem changes include swollen abdomen, a water-logged state of the carcase with fluid in the body cavities, under the skin and in the tissues generally. The liver is firm and swollen, with noticeably rounded edges and the heart may be enlarged and flabby. The lungs are dark and congested and the kidneys swollen. The gizzard is usually full of food. Mortality rarely exceeds 10 per cent and is often much less.

The cause of the condition is still unknown but there is no evidence of association with any infectious agent, nutritional factor or breed predisposition. There is some evidence that early management factors may be involved. Chilling or over-heating, over-crowding and the quantity of feed intake in the first few days may all be of some importance.

The characteristic post mortem changes are generally sufficient to establish a diagnosis, but confusion with round heart disease is possible and a heart condition due to feeding of **furazolidone**, which may give rise to similar post mortem changes, has been described. Continued feeding of furazolidone is necessary to produce this condition however and it is likely to be seen in older poults.

Little can be done by way of prevention of oedema syndrome other than careful attention to management and feeding.

HAEMORRHAGIC DISEASE

Nature and Incidence

This condition caused a good deal of alarm in the poultry industry of a decade or more ago because of its considerable incidence and the fact that the cause could not be determined. It has been reported as occurring throughout the U.S.A. and has been seen in a number of other countries including Britain. The condition is apparently less common today perhaps because a number of conditions in which haemorrhages occur, and which in earlier days were less well understood may have been grouped together and referred to as haemorrhagic disease. Infectious bursal disease, inclusion body hepatitis and gangrenous dermatitis are each characterised by haemorrhages in various organs or tissues and may at times have been included in the collective term haemorrhagic disease. No doubt however a separate entity also exists, the main finding in which is a haemorrhagic condition and the cause of which is still unknown.

Cause

A number of possible causes of the condition have been suggested over the years but none has yet been accepted as being responsible in every case. It is generally agreed, however, that in true haemorrhagic disease **no infectious agent is involved.** It is known that in many cases of haemorrhagic disease there is an association with the use of **sulphaquinoxaline** or other sulphonamides as **anti-coccidial agents.** It is believed that overdosing with these agents gives rise to a haemorrhagic disease, but that this is not a simple drug poisoning and that other unknown predisposing factors are necessary for clinical disease to result. **A deficiency of vitamin K,** a necessary agent for normal blood clotting, has also been suggested as a possible causative factor, but certain differences have been noted between haemorrhagic syndrome and vitamin K deficiency and the role of vitamin K in the disease is still uncertain.

Another possible causative agent in the condition is the presence of **preformed fungal toxins** in litter or food. These toxins are produced during growth of certain fungi in food or litter under favourable conditions of moisture and temperature. It has been shown experimentally that feeding of such toxins to chickens will give rise to a clinical condition with signs and post mortem changes similar to those of haemorrhagic syndrome. It may well be that ingestion of fungal toxins, or mycotoxicosis is one of the prime causes of the condition.

Signs

Haemorrhagic disease occurs mainly in chickens of four to eight weeks of age. Affected birds appear dejected, tend to huddle together with ruffled feathers and in some birds there is noticeable paleness of the comb and wattles. There may be diarrhoea with blood in the droppings and this may cause confusion with caecal coccidiosis. Mortality may be high or low, but in some cases the main clinical syndrome is inappetence, with poor food conversion and increased growing time being the main cause of economic loss.

Post mortem changes

Post mortem changes include pale bone marrow, watery blood, and haemorrhages of varying size in almost any organ or tissue particularly skin, muscular tissue, wall of intestine, gizzard and proventriculus, heart, liver, spleen and kidneys. There may be yellow or blood-stained fluid under the skin and in the body cavities.

Diagnosis of haemorrhagic disease must be based on the typical post mortem findings in conjunction with clinical signs in birds examined before death. It is essential to eliminate other known diseases in which haemorrhages are prominent before arriving at a diagnosis of haemorrhagic disease.

Treatment

Treatment of the condition will depend on circumstances in any particular case but, as a general rule, vitamin K has some beneficial effect due to its action in hastening blood clotting. In cases which occur during sulphonamide treatment for coccidiosis, it should be ensured that this is being used at the correct level and for the correct time. Overdosing or prolongation of treatment should be avoided. Where fungal toxins are suspected the source of these should be sought and removed where possible.

PULLET DISEASE

Nature and Incidence

A commonly diagnosed disease of pullets some years ago, pullet disease is rarely encountered at the present time. It was reported from a number of countries and was of considerable importance in America in the forties and fifties, occurring mainly in pullets coming into lay, although older and younger birds were sometimes affected. Cases also occurred in England. The disease was also called **avian monocytosis** because of the increased numbers of monocytes (one of the white cell series) in the blood. A disease of turkeys also called monocytosis, blue comb or transmissible enteritis occurs in Amerca, but is apparently unrelated to pullet disease.

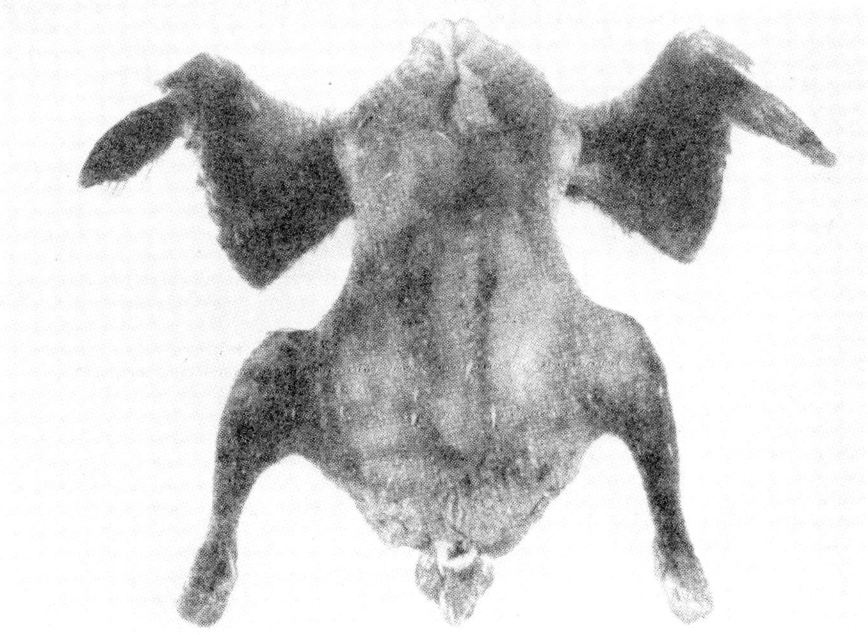

32.4 The most striking symptom of haemorrhagic disease is the moist nature of the carcase. In some areas, particularly of the wing, the skin appears to have liquified and a blood-stained fluid may ooze out.

Cause

The cause of pullet disease has never been fully established. It has been suggested that a virus is involved while other evidence indicated that it was a form of wheat poisoning. A sudden change of diet was also suggested as was poisoning by moulds in food. The disease apparently occurred more commonly in the summer months with a peak in July and August.

Signs

In a typical outbreak, many birds in a flock are suddenly noted to be ill. This sudden onset is quite characteristic. The main signs are inappetance, depression and a chalky white diarrhoea. Egg production falls sharply and a few dead birds may be picked up. The wattles and combs are darkened in colour and the eyes may appear sunken. Although appetite is depressed a common sign is a marked distension of the crop with a sour smelling fluid. Mortality may now increase and total losses may be as high as 50 per cent although 2 to 5 per cent is more usual.

The course of the disease usually extends over seven to ten days, most birds then recovering although several weeks may elapse before egg production returns to normal.

Post Mortem Changes
The main post mortem changes are dehydration, swelling and inflammation of the kidneys, urate deposits over the heart, liver and kidneys and degenerative changes in the ovaries of laying birds. Sour-crop, as mentioned earlier, will be found in many birds and staining of the tail feathers with chalky diarrhoea may be noticed.

Diagnosis of pullet disease is very much a case of careful observation of clinical signs and post mortem findings, and elimination of other diseases with similar clinical and post mortem features, particularly conditions involving the kidneys. There are no laboratory tests for the disease other than estimation of the number of monocytes in the blood, which is increased in typical cases.

Treatment
There is no specific treatment for the disease although claims have been made of good results following antibiotic treatment. Equally successful apparently has been addition of molasses to the drinking water. Probably one of the main aims of treatment should be provision of a plentiful supply of fresh water and avoidance of extremes of heat, cold or other stress.

PSITTACOSIS AND ORNITHOSIS

Nature and Incidence
Psittacosis is an infectious disease of psittacine birds (the parrot family) and man. The same condition in other birds is referred to as **ornithosis.** The disease is rare in birds in Britain but is of some importance in America particularly in turkeys, and in several other countries.

Cause
The disease is caused by an organism, *Chlamydia psittaci*, a member of the *Chlamydia* group which are related more closely to bacteria than to viruses. Members of the group cause a wide variety of diseases in man and animals.

Signs

In poultry, ornithosis causes a respiratory syndrome with general depression, ocular and nasal discharge, fast or difficult breathing, loss of appetite, greenish gelatinous diarrhoea and a severe drop in egg production. Mortality may be negligible or up to 30 per cent. Turkeys are usually more severely affected than chickens.

The source of infection in previously clean flocks is probably the droppings of wild birds. The organism survives in dried droppings for weeks or months and infection is acquired by inhalation of the organism in dust particles or possibly through skin wounds. Egg transmission does not occur.

Post Mortem Changes

Post mortem changes in birds which have died of ornithosis are seen mainly in the respiratory system and include lung congestion, pleuritic adhesions, fibrinous pericarditis, thickened cloudy air sacs and fluid in the chest cavity. The liver and spleen are enlarged and may show pin-point necrotic foci.

For a definite diagnosis of the condition, the signs and post mortem changes must be supported by microscopic examination of the liver and spleen either in histological sections or in impression smears of these organs. By special staining methods the organisms can be demonstrated as minute intracellular particles or inclusions. Additional serological and biological tests may also be used.

Treatment

Treatment with **chlortetracycline** is effective in controlling clinical disease but prolonged treatment is required and total elimination of the organism from infected birds is not necessarily achieved. Recovered carrier birds are important in perpetuating the infection in a flock. Thorough cleaning and disinfection of premises following an outbreak is essential. The **possibility and danger of transmission of the disease to humans must be borne in mind** and every precaution taken when handling infected carcases and dealing with outbreaks.

CANNIBALISM & FEATHER PECKING

This is a common vice rather than a disease which in some flocks can reach epidemic proportions and result in considerable economic loss. The condition is commoner in light bodied, white breeds than heavy brown types and is more serious in birds in cages than on litter. It is rarely seen in broilers.

The degree of damage inflicted varies from slight feather pecking to complete pecking out of the intestines through the vent. When the condition starts in a cage house it often rapidly escalates, birds seemingly developing a pecking habit which can be extremely difficult to break. Birds at the lower end of the pecking order are attacked by their more dominant companions and are unable to escape in the confines of the cage.

Causes

There are a number of possible causes of the condition. There may be an inherited tendency in some breeds, particularly the light "flighty" type. Overcrowding of birds in cages or on litter will predispose to cannibalism as will insufficient trough space per bird. Over-bright lighting is often accompanied by cannibalism and sheer boredom may well be a potent causative factor. It is doubtful if dietary deficiencies or external parasites are of much significance in the condition but one other likely precipitating factor is a high incidence of prolapse of oviduct sometimes seen in flocks approaching peak production or in immature birds which have been brought to lay too early.

Prevention

Prevention of the vice depends on avoidance of managerial factors which may precipitate it. Reduced light intensity by means of a dimmer mechanism or use of red coloured bulbs, avoidance of overstocking, ensuring adequate trough space, feeding of mash rather than pellets to layers (as is almost universally done nowadays) in order to give the birds a degree of preoccupation and so avoid boredom, all have their part to play. The most positive measure however is **debeaking** of the flock at a convenient time during rearing. Cannibalism is seldom a serious problem in birds which have been correctly debeaked.

When a severe outbreak occurs in a laying flock lowering the light intensity usually gives a measure of control. Debeaking of birds in lay is seldom practical. Application of **Stockholm tar** to wounds on pecked birds acts as an antiseptic dressing and as a repellent to attacking birds. Various other substances in the form of sprays, lotions, etc., have been used but their value is doubtful.

GIZZARD EROSION

This is a condition of the gizzard of broiler chickens in which the inner lining of the gizzard becomes eroded by crater-like lesions which penetrate the lining, often with an accompanying dark discoloration of the gizzard and its contents.

The cause of the condition is uncertain but dietary factors are believed to be involved, particularly a high level of fish meal in the food. No mortality is caused, but there is apparently some reduction in weight gain of affected birds. One of the most important effects of gizzard erosion however is the fact that gizzards are rendered unmarketable, or made difficult to process for human consumption.

No completely effective treatment is known, but **additional Vitamin E** appears to have some beneficial effect.

TUMOURS

The vast majority of the tumours found in chickens are those associated with leucosis and lymphomatosis. Other tumours do occur, although it is difficult to obtain exact information as to their incidence and the losses they cause in view of the difficulty in differentiating them from the various manifestations of leucosis and lymphomatosis. That they do occur, however, is certain, as is the fact that they present no great problem to the poultry industry.

Like the tumours that affect other animals, they can be classified into those that do not spread within the body (benign) and those that do (malignant). They usually occur in mature birds, and may be found in all the various systems of the body. The blood circulatory system is by no means exempt, the so-called "bleeding cyst," well recognised by poultry farmers, being an example.

CHEMICAL POISONS

Under modern methods of management chemical poisoning of poultry is a fairly rare event, much rarer than many poultry farmers suspect if one can judge from the information supplied with dead birds submitted to laboratories for post-mortem examination.

The poisoning of poultry that does occur is usually due to accident or carelessness in the use of drugs and chemicals as medicinal agents, for the control of vermin around poultry premises, or for horticultural purposes. The need for employing drugs in the treatment of poultry disease exactly according to the manufacturers' instructions has been stressed in previous chapters; it cannot be over-emphasised.

Apart from drugs used in the treatment of avian disease, the chemicals most commonly implicated in poisoning include phosphorus and zinc phosphide in rat poisons, and mercury, nicotine, arsenic, and more recently developed agents like aldrin, in horticultural preparations, seed dressings, etc.

The symptoms exhibited by poisoned birds are not usually sufficiently characteristic to indicate that the birds, in fact, have been poisoned, let alone to indicate the particular poison involved. Nor are the changes found in the internal organs during a post-mortem examination. However, poisoning may be considered a possibility when a number of birds in a flock suddenly become ill or die and when no other cause can be found to account for the trouble experienced.

It is helpful, if not essential, for poultry farmers who suspect poisoning in their flocks to supply information regarding any particular poison to which their birds might have been exposed when submitting carcases to a diagnostic laboratory, since only in exceptional circumstances can these laboratories carry out examinations for the presence of poisons in general.

APPENDIX

GLOSSARY OF MEDICAL TERMS

Agglutination   clumping; usually of blood cells or micro–organisms.

Alimentary   referring to the digestive tract.

Antibody   a substance produced as part of the body's immune response to invasion by an antigen. Its function is to render the antigen harmless.

Antigen   a chemical substance or micro–organism which when introduced into the body gives rise to the production of antibodies by the animal's immune mechanisms.

Asphyxiation   suffocation.

Atrophy   wasting; often accompanied by a reduction in size of an organ or tissue.

Attenuate   to reduce the disease causing ability, usually of a micro–organism.

Caecal tubes   the blind guts; a pair of blind–ending appendages of the intestine.

Capillaries   the smallest blood vessels.

Carrier   an animal which is infected by, and may excrete, an organism without itself showing signs of disease or ill-health.

Caseous   cheese–like.

Chronic   having a prolonged course; of disease or inflammation.

Cloaca   the vent.

Commensal   an animal or organism which lives on or in another species without causing it any injury or harm.

Congestion   increased flow of blood to an organ or tissue resulting in reddening of the part.

Conjunctivitis   inflammation of the conjunctiva or lining membrane of the eye socket.

Dehydrated   dried out; excessively dry, of the body of tissues.

Duodenum   the first part of the small intestine immediately following the gizzard.

Endemic   constantly present in a country or area.

Enteritis   inflammation of the intestine.

Epidemic   a sudden outbreak of a rapidly spreading disease in an area.

Epithelium   the outermost layer of skin or mucous membrane.

Exudate   material, usually fluid together with cells and other debris, which is deposited in tissues or body cavities as a result of its escape from blood vessels in the course of the inflammatory response.

Fibrin   a protein of the blood, sometimes deposited in the tissues in the course of certain diseases.

Flocculent   containing solid particles or masses.

Friable   soft with a tendency to disintegrate; usually of the liver.

Growth plate   the region near the end of a long bone where growth takes place.

Hepatitis   inflammation of the liver.

Histology   the study of tissues, particularly as seen under the microscope.

Hock joint   the joint at the junction of the feathered and unfeathered parts of the leg.

Hormone   a chemical substance produced by one of a number of glands in the body and released into the blood stream to influence another organ.

Impaction   obstruction of a hollow organ by a contained physical mass.

Inactivated   killed; usually refers to micro–organisms particularly those contained in a vaccine.

Inappetance   lack of appetite.

Incidence   the degree of prevalence of a disease in a country or area.

Inclusion Body   an aggregation of virus particles visible microscopically in certain cells in some viral diseases.

Incubation period   the interval of time which must elapse between the picking up of an infectious or parasitic disease and the animal first showing signs of disease.

Ingestion   eating; taking of food or other material by mouth.

Inspissated   thickened, solidified.

Isolation   the culture of organisms in the laboratory, usually from a case of disease or contaminated environment.

Lesion   an abnormality of any kind in any organ or tissue, which may be visible grossly or microscopically.

Lumen   the internal cavity of a hollow organ such as the intestine.

Lymphocyte   one of the white cells of the blood, whose main function is concerned with immunity.

Lymphoid   referring to the lymphocytes.

Metabolism   the sum of all the chemical and physical processes which proceed within the body in life.

Monocyte   one of the white blood cells.

Mucous membrane   the lining membrane of the internal hollow organs such as the intestine, blood vessels, windpipe etc.

Necrosis   death of tissue.

Necrotic foci   small areas of necrosis, usually visible as yellow–white spots in an organ or tissue and often occurring in the course of an infection.

Nephrotoxic   having the ability to damage the kidneys.

Neoplasia   "new growth", tumour formation, cancer.

Neural, neurological   referring to the nerves or nervous system.

Neutralising   a term applied to a type of antibody.

Nodule   a small, solid mass in an organ or tissue.

Oedema   an abnormal accumulation of fluid in an organ, tissue or body cavity.

Oesophagus   the gullet, the tube down which food passes from the throat to the stomach.

Oral   by mouth.

Oviduct   the tube in which the albumen and shell of the egg are added to the yolk and which conveys the egg to the vent.

Parboiled   having a partly cooked appearance.
Pathogen   a disease–causing agent.
Pathogenic   having the ability to cause disease.
Pericardium   the thin transparent membrane which surrounds and encloses the heart.
Pericarditis   inflammation of the pericardium.
Peritonitis   inflammation of the peritoneum or lining membrane of the abdominal cavity.
Plexus   a network of vessels or nerves.
Poult   a young turkey or pheasant.
Precipitating   refers to a type of antibody.
Protozoa   microscopic organisms, the lowest form of animal life. Some are disease–causing parasites.
Proventriculus   the true stomach of the fowl, situated between the oesophagus and the gizzard.
Purulent   containing or composed of pus.
Pustule   a small pus-filled eruption in the skin or mucous membrane.
Sabourauds medium   a laboratory medium used for culture of fungi.
Septicaemia   a severe stage of infectious disease in which vast numbers of organisms enter the blood stream. It is accompanied by fever, severe generalised illness and often results in death.
Serotype   the type of a micro–organism according to its antigenic structure.
Sinus   a hollow space or cavity. Usually refers to the air space in the bones of the nose and face.
Subclinical   with no visible signs of disease.
Subcutaneous   under the skin.
Thoracic   referring to or within the chest.
Titre   the amount of one substance which reacts with another. Usually refers to the degree of positiveness of a blood test.
Toxaemia   blood poisoning, usually due to absorption of bacterial toxins from a site of infection.
Toxin   poison. In this book usually refers to a poison of bacterial origin.
Toxic   poisonous.
Ulcer   a break in the continuity of skin or mucous membrane.
Urates   white, chalk–like material normally excreted by the kidneys, but deposited in abnormal situations in the bird's body in certain disease states.
Ureters   the tubes which convey urine from the kidneys to the vent.
Vector   a mechanical carrier or transmitter of disease.
Vesicle   a small blister.
Virulence   the degree of ability to cause disease.

Index

240

241